Download Ebook

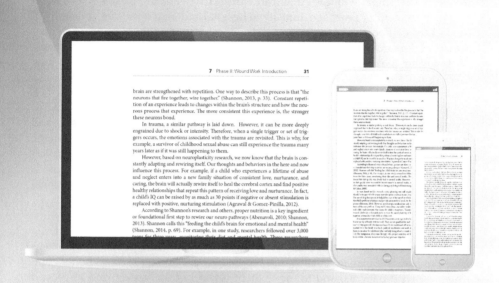

Your print purchase of *CMSA's Integrated Case Management*
includes an ebook download to the device of your choice—
increasing accessibility, portability, and searchability!

Download your ebook today at
http://spubonline.com/cmsa
and enter the access code below:

FT6RWHEW

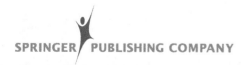

SPRINGER PUBLISHING COMPANY

Kathleen Fraser, MSN, MHA, RN-BC, CCM, CRRN, has been a registered nurse since 1980. She holds two master's degrees, one from Texas A & M University and the second and most recent from St. Joseph's College, Standish, Maine. Ms. Fraser is a certified case manager, a certified rehabilitation registered nurse, and is board certified in case management with the American Nurses Credentialing Center. She entered case management 24 years ago, initially in hospital and long-term care, then moved to workers' compensation for 21 years. Ms. Fraser served on the Case Management Society of America's (CMSA's) National Board of Directors, holding four positions, the last being the office of national president (from 2014 through 2016), then became CMSA's national executive director immediately following her presidency. She also became a master trainer for CMSA's Integrated Case Management program, which led to this manual. She has served on numerous case management panels, boards, councils, foundations, and committees, in the United States and internationally, and is a noted case management author and speaker. Kathleen has received many awards, including being selected by Seak, Inc., and the National Workers' Compensation and Occupational Medicine Conference as one of the "50 Most Influential People in Workers' Compensation and Occupational Medicine," and the 2016 CMSA National Case Manager of the Year award.

Rebecca Perez, BSN, RN, CCM, has a bachelor's degree in nursing and is a certified case manager with extensive clinical and case management experience. Much of her case management career has been spent honing skills to better communicate with patients, and to move them toward self-advocacy and improved health outcomes. She has been involved with the Case Management Society of America (CMSA) since 1997, holding both local and national leadership positions and honored with the 2013 National CMSA Case Manager of the Year award. She is a published author of professional articles, Case Management Adherence Guidelines and a coauthor of the 2010 *Integrated Case Management Manual*. Ms. Perez was a developer of CMSA's Integrated Case Management training curriculum and was a master trainer for the program. She has created CMSA's new Integrated Case Management Training Program to coincide with this manual, providing advanced practical skills and training to case managers working with individuals with health complexity. Ms. Perez recently moved into the position as director of product development for Fraser Imagineers and the CMSA. She also serves as the executive director for the CMSA Case Management Foundation.

Corine Latour, PhD, RN, graduated in 1987 from the Amsterdam University of Applied Sciences Faculty of Health/School of Nursing. After graduating, she worked in the field of psychiatry and specialized in consultation and liaison psychiatry at the Free University Medical Centre, Amsterdam, Netherlands. During this period, she earned her PhD. The subject of her thesis was "Coordination of Care for the Complex Medically Ill." Dr. Latour is the director of the School of Nursing at the University of Applied Sciences, Amsterdam, Netherlands. She is an associate professor for integrated psychiatric and somatic care at the university and is a contributor to the development of integrated case management in partnership with the Case Management Society of America (CMSA). Dr. Latour is a board member of the INTERMED Foundation, board member of the National Nursing Education Organization (LOOV), a core member of the Nurse Science and Innovation Center (NSI) Amsterdam and a published author.

CMSA's Integrated Case Management

A Manual for Case Managers by Case Managers

Kathleen Fraser, *MSN, MHA, RN-BC, CCM, CRRN*

Rebecca Perez, *BSN, RN, CCM*

Corine Latour, *PhD, RN*

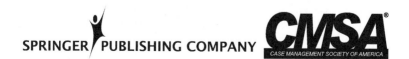

SPRINGER PUBLISHING COMPANY

Springer Publishing Company, LLC
11 West 42nd Street
New York, NY 10036
www.springerpub.com

Acquisitions Editor: Elizabeth Nieginski
Senior Production Editor: Kris Parrish
Compositor: S4Carlisle Publishing Services

ISBN: 978-0-8261-6941-9
ebook ISBN: 978-0-8261-6951-8
18 19 20 21 / 6 5 4 3 2

Library of Congress Cataloging-in-Publication Data

Names: Fraser, Kathleen (Registered nurse), author. | Perez, Rebecca, author.
   | Latour, Corine, author. | Case Management Society of America.
Title: CMSA's integrated case management : a manual for case managers by case
   managers / Kathleen Fraser, Rebecca Perez, Corine Latour.
Other titles: Case Management Society of America's integrated case management
   | Integrated case management
Description: New York : Springer Publishing Company, [2018] | Includes
   bibliographical references and index.
Identifiers: LCCN 2017049619 | ISBN 9780826169419
Subjects: | MESH: Case Management--organization & administration | Delivery
   of Health Care, Integrated--organization & administration | Case Managers
   | Professional Role
Classification: LCC RA971 | NLM W 84.7 | DDC 362.1068--dc23 LC record available at
   https://lccn.loc.gov/2017049619

"In a gentle way you can shake the world."
—*Mahatma Gandhi*

Contents

PART IV: Transitions of Care and Accreditation Care in Integrated Case Management

Foreword

Case managers, in concert with other health care professionals, have difficulty meeting individual and family health care needs due to the propensity for managing chronic behavioral health conditions in isolation from a patient's chronic medical condition. This silo case management process followed the medical model of treating a patient's disease, rather than treating an individual holistically with all components of his or her disease and health taken under consideration. Case managers embrace the population health model, and the opportunity to meet the triple aim—improving the patient experience of care (including quality and satisfaction); improving the health of populations; and reducing the per capita cost of health care.

The Case Management Society of America (CMSA) has long been an advocate for an integrated approach to patient and client case management services because it provides the best outcomes for patients, clients, soldiers, and veterans. However, the infrastructure and tools are not readily available to case managers to provide comprehensive case management services.

The initial *Integrated Case Management (ICM) Manual* addressed this need from a global and interprofessional perspective. Case managers will find in the new ICM manual a focused guide, written specifically by and for case managers on how to assess an individual, and together create a case management plan, designed with the individual's goals at the center of the plan. The steps for the identified interventions and the necessary evaluation of long- and short-term goals are clearly defined in the new manual. The case manager has the opportunity to review the ICM tool and selected case studies that map the patient/client–centered plan of care for the achievement of both short- and long-term goals.

The CMSA Standards of Practice (SOP) incorporate the patient advocate role as fundamental to all other standards. ICM is the method that embraces the value of patient advocacy and allows the patient to determine his or her goals and the actions necessary to achieve these goals. The case manager is the trusted partner in assisting with plan and goal development and with the process of evaluating and adjusting the plan to achieve a value-based outcome.

The case manager using the ICM model has the ability to assess a patient's or client's historical and current socioeconomic risks in conjunction with the medical, cognitive, and behavioral risks. This comprehensive model addresses unresolved past issues and problems with a patient's and client's current challenges. The ICM approach also seeks to mitigate risk and prevent future setbacks or catastrophic events.

It is my great honor to present this new ICM manual written by my CMSA case manager colleagues for all case managers across the care continuum.

Mary McLaughlin Davis, DNP, MSN, ACNS-BC, NEA-BC, CCM
2016–2018 CMSA National President
Little Rock, Arkansas

Preface

It is my honor, as CMSA's executive director, to introduce *CMSA's Integrated Case Management* written by case managers for case managers. It is intended to bring to case managers a relevant textbook to enable the care transition processes of integration, which are safe and well-coordinated. The format is more conducive to individualization per organization, making the process not only attainable but easily and readily usable, irrespective of the setting or genre. This reference manual for nurses and other health professionals presents a CMSA-tested approach toward systematically integrating physical and mental health case management principles and assessment tools. The health care field has undergone major changes and health care workers must know how to integrate those new regulations, describe alternative payment options, and implement requirements for greater patient and family assessment, care planning, and care coordination into their practice.

Through collaboration, we can reduce duplications in health care, avoid gaps, and reduce health care costs—this is the essence of case management. It involves continual communication with patients, their caregivers, and the various professionals and services with which they come into contact. Fundamental to the collaboration is the presence of the case manager, taking the responsibility for overseeing and coordinating that care and helping patients and caregivers to navigate the system. This navigational role is important, because most individuals selected for case management need services or input from one or more providers. The cumulative impact of multiple strategies (rather than single interventions) is more likely to be successful in improving patient experiences and case management outcomes; therefore, it should be one of the key tools that is part of a wider strategy for integrated care.

CMSA's Integrated Case Management delves into the role of the case manager and unpacks how case managers assess and treat complex patients. These are patients who may be challenged with medical and behavioral conditions, poor access to care services, as well as chronic illnesses and disabilities, and require multidisciplinary care to regain health and function. With a wealth of information on regulatory requirements, new models of care, integration of services, digital and telemedicine, and new performance measures that are clearly defined for nurses in nursing terminology, chapters outline the steps needed to begin, implement, and use the interventions of the integrated case management approach. As a coauthor of the manual, I was thrilled that we were able to align all content with the newly revised 2017 Model Care Act, the CMSA Standards of Practice 2016 as well as the *CMSA Core Curriculum for Case Management*, Third Edition. By integrating the concepts and proven practice foundations of case management, your patients can truly benefit by utilizing the integration of behavioral health and physical health, using treatment guidelines and risk stratification methods created by case managers for *you*, the case manager!

Kathleen Fraser

Acknowledgments

The authors would like to acknowledge and express their sincere gratitude to the following professionals for their invaluable contributions to the development of this manual:

Jos Dobber, MSc, RN
Amsterdam University of Applied Sciences
For content development in the chapter on motivational interviewing

Deborah Gutteridge, MS, CBIST
Regional Manager of Marketing and Business Development-Central, NeuroRestorative
For providing evidence and consultation regarding traumatic brain injury

Paul Ciechanowski, MD, MPH
Founder/Chief Medical Officer, Samepage, Inc.
For providing research and support demonstrating the value of an integrated approach

Mary McLaughlin Davis, DNP, MSN, ACNS-BC, NEA-BC, CCM
CMSA National President 2016–2018
Special appreciation to Dr. McLaughlin Davis for the support provided in the development of this manual and unlimited commitment to the practice and power of case management.

PART I

Introduction to Integrated Case Management and Its Models

CHAPTER 1

The Evolution of Case Management and the Professional Case Manager

Kathleen Fraser

Rebecca Perez

I have an almost complete disregard of precedent, and a faith in the possibility of something better. It irritates me to be told how things have always been done. I defy the tyranny of precedent. I go for anything new that might improve the past.

—Clara Barton

OBJECTIVES

- Understand the evolution of case management
- Understand the new 2016 *Standards of Practice for Case Management*
- Understand professional case management roles, functions, activities, and responsibilities
- Understand how evidence-based practice is demonstrated

As early as the 19th century, charitable organizations were providing services to persons in need, an undertaking which predated any organized government role in the delivery of human services. The oldest genre of formal case management is that of workers' compensation. Workers' compensation legislation was enacted in 1911 and case management soon followed. In 1943, Liberty Mutual used in-house case management as a cost management measure for workers' compensation insurance. The first workers' compensation case managers were rehabilitation nurses and vocational specialists. Their jobs were and remain as coordinators of care for the injured worker to return safely to gainful employment in the highest level of physical and mental health, medically possible. The case manager works with not only the injured worker (patient), the treating physician, all specialists, therapists, and any other members of the care team as well as the employer and the claims adjuster. Care coordination and early intervention is critical to ensure that the injured worker receives the medical care needed to address conditions in a timely manner.

A significant impact of the development of organized services occurred with the Social Security Act (SSA) of 1932. It not only established a major role for the federal government in meeting human needs, the SSA attempted to bring together programs such as public assistance, maternal social insurance, and child health. The result was a delivery system compartmentalized into separate bureaucracies. Post-World War II, insurance companies employed nurses and social workers to assist with the coordination of care for soldiers returning from the war who suffered complex injuries requiring multidisciplinary intervention. Many nurses were employed as case managers to help returning wounded veterans receive multiple interventions required as part of their rehabilitation. To date, this remains a significant area of practice with case managers playing an integral role for our military returning to a "normal life" post battlefield injuries. The case managers exponentially increased the chance of successful outcomes.

In 1962, the President's Panel on Mental Retardation proposed the "continuum of care" as a critical consideration. This concept would later evolve into what is now called "case management." The Developmental Disabilities Act of 1975 established case management as a "priority service." Critical attempts were made to establish programs that would integrate services, and these programs became the forerunners of case management. The term "services integration" was coined to describe federally initiated activities that attempted to build linkages among human service programs and bring coordination to the social service system. The current delivery of case management services is derived from the fragmented and duplicative efforts of these early, singular organizations and legislation.

By the mid-1980s, health insurers developed case management programs targeted at the catastrophically injured and ill population. There were double-digit inflation rates for medical costs moving the focus on cost containment. During this time, as they had from the beginning, nurses, social workers, and all other case management disciplines worked without standards of practice certifying what exactly constituted case management.

Concurrently, spiraling health care costs with diminishing revenues and reimbursement made hospitals particularly challenged to focus on patient length of stay, early discharge, and management of costs. The proliferation and the increased cost of services, the complexity of the service system multiplied for all types of persons with long-term care needs, strategy regarding coordination of services, also left large deficits in state Medicaid budgets forcing many state budget personnel to seek ways to control costs. Hence, case management has been viewed as a key element in cost control, not only patient advocacy. This increasing demand for health care services created a crisis in health care delivery along with a crisis of enormously increasing Medicaid expenditures for nursing home care for their elderly citizens with the factor of 80% of the elderly experiencing chronic illnesses.

In 1995, the Case Management Society of America (CMSA) became the first organization to develop *Standards of Practice for Case Management*. These standards allowed those in the practice to demonstrate to physicians, payers, legislators, and other members of the health care team exactly what the practice of case management entailed. These *Standards of Practice* made it possible for any organization, no matter the genre, that employs case managers, to build policies and procedures that ensure their organizations are compliant with the requirements established by licensing bodies and accreditation organizations. They were revised in 2010 and most recently in 2016.

The CMSA 2016 Standards of Practice *states:*

"Case Management is a collaborative process of assessment, planning, facilitation, care coordination, evaluation and advocacy for options and services to meet an individual's and family's comprehensive health needs through communication and available resources to promote patient safety, quality of care, and cost effective outcomes."

The impetus for the 2016 revision of the *Standards of Practice for Case Management* was the need to emphasize the professional nature of the practice and the role of the case manager. The maturity of the practice of case management and the importance of protecting the professional role of case managers legitimize professional case management as an integral and necessary component of the health care delivery system. The 2016 *Standards of Practice for Case Management* are meant to communicate the value of professional case management practice to:

- Update the *definition of case management* to reflect recent changes in the practice.
- Clarify who the *professional case manager* is and the qualifications expected of this professional.
- Emphasize the practice of *professional case management* in the ever-expanding care settings across the entire continuum of health and human services, and in constant collaboration with the client, the client's family or family caregiver, and members of the interprofessional health care team.
- Communicate *practical expectations* of professional case managers in the application of each standard. These are found in the "how demonstrated" section that follows each standard.
- Reflect legislative and regulatory changes affecting professional case management practice such as the need to include the *client's family* or family *caregiver* in the provision of case management services and to the client's satisfaction.
- Replace the use of stigmatizing terms such as "problems" and "issues" with others that are empowering to the client such as "care needs" and "opportunities."
- Communicate the *"closure"* of case management services and the case manager–client relationship instead of *"termination"* of services and/or the case management process. This subtle change is better reflective of the reality that despite case closure, a client may continue to receive health care services, however not in a case management context.
- Emphasize the provision of *client-centered* and *culturally* and *linguistically appropriate* case management services.
- Highlight the *value of professional case management* practice and the role of the professional case manager.
- Recognize the need for professional case managers to engage in *scholarly activities*, including research, evidence-based practice (EBP), performance improvement and innovation, and lifelong learning.

FIGURE 1.1 The Continuum of Health Care and Professional Case Management model (CMSA, 2016).

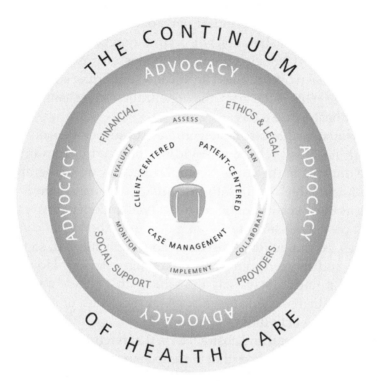

Source: Case Management Society of America (2016).

Professional Case Management Roles, Functions, Activities, and Responsibilities

As stated in the 2016 *CMSA Standards of Practice*, "It is necessary to differentiate between the terms 'role,' 'function,' and 'activity' before describing the responsibilities of professional case managers. Defining these terms provides a clear and contextual understanding of the roles and responsibilities of case managers in the various practice settings." The standards illustrate why we are the recognized experts and vital participants in the care coordination team. The standards stress we empower people to understand and access quality, efficient health care. It recognizes our worth as financial stewards and our ability to work with all stakeholders, yet stresses in times of ethical conflict, patient advocacy always comes first. They lay out the ethical standards of care we practice and serve to support the case management profession. Most case management companies and/or departments use or address these standards as their basis for policy. Case management is neither linear nor a one-way exercise. Facilitation, coordination, and collaboration will occur throughout the client's health care encounter. Collaboration among physicians, pharmacists, nurses, case managers, social workers, allied health and supporting staff is critical in achieving the goals of the team, the organization, and changing the way we deliver health care today.

The awareness that case managers are crucial members of the health care team has been realized providing the need to reexamine and redefine our role in the current complex health care topography. The body of knowledge required to practice case management is rapidly growing as the specialty continues to evolve. Modern patient care must be based on the holistic intertwining of information from a variety of disciplines. As our activities become more sophisticated, so must our resources and those resources must remain relevant. However, the one area that must always stay the same is that we are patient advocates. Our patients/clients are always at the center of *all* our shared decision-making activities (see Figure 1.1).

A "role" is a general and abstract term that refers to a set of behaviors and expected consequences that are associated with one's position in a social structure. A "function" is a grouping or a set of specific tasks or activities within the role. An "activity" is a discrete action, behavior, or task a person performs to address the expectations of the role assumed. A role consists of several functions and each function is described through a list of specific and related activities. These descriptions constitute what is commonly known as a "job description."

The case management process is a set of steps applied by case managers to their approach to patient care management. It is similar to the nursing process or problem-solving approaches; however, the process of case management is practiced in virtually every setting across the continuum and is much broader than the nursing process alone. The case management process is a systemic approach to patient care delivery and management. The case manager works closely with various members of the interdisciplinary health care team in implementing the case management process and interventions. It cannot happen in isolation of the contributions of other health care professionals. Thus, case management practice is a team approach. Case managers are constantly collaborating and coordinating the client's care and services with other health care providers. Regardless of the type of team, it is always important to include the client and client's support system as part of the team. The team exists because of the client and the team's goals are what the client/support system agrees upon. The team is then able to provide client-centered care.

The professional case manager performs the primary functions of assessment, planning, facilitation, coordination, monitoring, evaluation, and advocacy. Integral to these functions are collaboration and ongoing communication with the client, the client's family or family caregiver, and other health care professionals involved in the client's care. Performing the initial full assessment of the client/patient encompasses his or her health, physical, functional, behavioral, psychological, and social needs, including health literacy status and deficits. Self-management abilities and engagement in taking care of one's own health, availability of psychosocial support systems including family caregivers, and socioeconomic background are also captured. Because the client/patient is always at the center of all care plans, the case manager strives to promote client self-advocacy, independence, and self-determination, and the provision of client-centered and culturally appropriate care. Assessment begins next and involves data gathering, analysis, and synthesis of information for developing a client-centered integrated case management plan of care. It helps establish the client–case manager's relationship and the client's readiness to engage in his or her own health and well-being. It requires the use of effective communication skills such as active listening, meaningful conversation, motivational interviewing, and use of open-ended questions.

Care needs and opportunities are identified through analysis of the assessment findings and determination of identified needs, barriers, and/or gaps in care. Note that the case management process is cyclical and recurrent, rather than linear and unidirectional. For example, key functions of the professional case manager occur throughout all the steps of the case management process by remaining in constant contact with the client, caregiver, and other members of the interprofessional health care team. Primary steps in the case management process include screening clients identified or referred by other professionals for case management to determine appropriateness for, and benefits from, services and then obtaining consent for case management services as part of the case initiation process.

The philosophy of case management underscores the recommendation that at-risk individuals, especially those with complex medical, behavioral, and/or psychosocial needs, be evaluated for case management intervention. The key philosophical components of case management address care that is holistic and client centered, with mutual goals, allowing stewardship of resources for the client and the health care system including the diverse group of stakeholders. Through these efforts, case management focuses simultaneously on achieving optimal health and attaining wellness to the highest level possible for each client. Case managers use their understanding of illness or injury, treatments, and the components of care that may serve as barriers to improvement by impeding care from the client's providers. Integrated case management interventions reduce the fragmentation of services recipients of care often experience when multiple health care providers include behavioral health issues and needs. When the provision of health care is effective and efficient, all parties benefit. Case management, fully integrating the medical and behavioral needs of the individual, serves to identify options and resources that are acceptable to the client and client's family or caregiver. This in turn increases the potential for effective client engagement in self-management, adherence to the case management plan of care, and the achievement of successful outcomes.

For professional case managers, delivery of care is accomplished through a network of resources. Whether case managers work in a hospital or other acute-care setting, for an insurer or third-party provider or in another venue, identifying the appropriate resources is at the heart of advocacy for patients. Now, as new models of care delivery continue to emerge, the professional case manager—particularly one who is board-certified—will be at the heart of these networks to coordinate care, facilitate communication, and employ evidence-based practice (EBP) in pursuit of positive outcomes (Boshier, 2011). Amid these new complexities in care delivery, primary care physicians must either try to do everything themselves—which while effective, is not efficient—or they must hire case managers whose roles and responsibilities are integrated into their care. Therein lies the challenge for primary care physicians, who may not be familiar with the roles and functions of a case manager. Physicians who have limited knowledge of case management could erroneously utilize nonclinical staff for case management duties. Although nonclinical staff can be used for duties such as paperwork processing, use of these individuals to address patient needs is inappropriate and could expose the physician to liability.

Case management also involves speaking up when organizational leadership proposes such actions in a misdirected effort to maximize available resources while minimizing the costs of professional staffing. It is essential to help business leaders understand that undermining the role of the professional case manager in this way jeopardizes patient safety, fractures coordinated care, and weakens quality outcomes. Only professional case managers, by their licensing, can perform a full patient assessment that may include:

Medical

- Presenting health status and conditions
- Medical history including use of prescribed or over-the-counter medications and herbal therapies
- Relevant treatment history
- Prognosis
- Nutritional status

Cognitive and behavioral

- Mental health
    - History of substance use
    - Depression risk screening
    - History of treatment including prescribed or over-the-counter medications and herbal therapies
- Cognitive functioning
    - Language and communication preferences, needs, or limitations
- Client strengths and abilities
    - Self-care and self-management capability
    - Readiness to change
- Client professional and educational focus
    - Vocational and/or educational interests
    - Recreational and leisure pursuits
- Self-management and engagement status
    - Health literacy
    - Health activation level

- Knowledge of health condition
- Knowledge of and adherence to plan of care
- Medication management and adherence
- Learning and technology capabilities

Social

- Psychosocial status
    - Family or family caregiver dynamics
    - Caregiver resources: availability and degree of involvement
    - Environmental and residential
- Financial circumstances
- Client beliefs, values, needs, and preferences including cultural and spiritual
- Access to care
    - Health insurance status and availability of health care benefits
    - Health care providers involved in care of clients
    - Barriers to getting care and resources
- Safety concerns and needs
    - History of neglect, abuse, violence, or trauma
    - Safety of the living situation
- Advanced directives planning and availability of documentation
- Pertinent legal situations (e.g., custody, marital discord, and immigration status)

Functional

- Client priorities and self-identified care goals
- Functional status
- Transitional or discharge planning needs and services, if applicable

- Health care services currently or recently received in the home setting
- Skilled nursing, home health aide, durable medical equipment (DME), or other relevant services
- Transportation capability and constraints
- Follow-up care (e.g., primary care, specialty care, and appointments)
- Safety and appropriateness of home or residential environment
- Reassessment of the client's condition, response to the case management plan of care and interventions, and progress toward achieving care goals and target outcomes
- Documentation of resource utilization and cost management, provider options, and available health and behavioral care benefits
- Evidence of relevant information and data required for the client's thorough assessment and obtained from multiple sources including, but not limited to:
  - Client interviews
  - Initial and ongoing assessments and care summaries available in the client's health record and across the transitions of care
  - Family caregivers (as appropriate), physicians, providers, and other involved members of the interprofessional health care team
  - Past medical records available as appropriate
  - Claims and administrative data

For more information on nonlicensed/noncertified personnel, please refer to Chapter 9.

Evidence-Based Practice

Evidence-based practice (EBP) means integrating the individual case manager's clinical expertise with the best available external clinical *evidence* from systematic research. This should be obtained through expert opinions, practice analyses, and roles and functions research following evidence-based guidelines while considering predictive modeling. Then to put into practice, the case manager integrates the two aspects of clinical expertise and clinical evidence with the individual patient's own values. This implementation into all aspects of the shared decision-making processes will yield a full comprehensive assessment and a subsequent professional case management service of care toward the goal of positive outcomes. In the *Professional Case Management* journal, editor Suzanne Powell writes: "Evidence-based guidelines are becoming essential tools in the practice of case management. They serve as that valued resource that allows the individual case manager to be proactive in planning, educating the patient and the multidisciplinary team" (Powell, 2008). Evidence-based case management does not rely on opinions but on actual evidence examination. Evidence enhances our practice by providing additional tools needed for the case manager to ensure the delivery of safe, quality care.

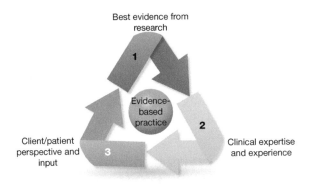

So why do case managers shy away from EBP utilization?

Excuses given:

- Hard to access research articles
- Difficulty understanding, interpreting, implementing into practice
- Too little time to research
- Lack of confidence in how to find the research findings needed

However, the failure to integrate the principles of EBP into our daily practice prevents our practice from moving forward as a profession. Utilization of EBP into integrated case management need not be difficult. First ask yourself, what is an issue you need resolved? Then search online for related evidence applicable to your issue. Analyze the source as to its significance and analytical testing and if that evidence supports practice change. If you and your team decide to utilize it, it can lead to valuable improvement initiatives for not only case managers but for the organization as well. This is how change can occur and who better to be a change agent than a case manager?

CMSA Model Care Act

According to the 2017 Model Care Act, professional case managers are health care professionals and pioneers of health care change. They serve as health care team leaders who open new areas of thought and research and development. Professional case managers positively impact and improve consumer well-being and health care outcomes. Professional case management roles and functions lead to quality care and successful outcomes. Such outcomes cannot be achieved without the specialized skills, knowledge, and competencies professional case managers apply throughout the case management process. Professional case manager competencies include critical thinking and analysis, motivational interviewing, effective communication, positive relationship building, ability to plan and organize effectively, negotiation, cost-conscious allocation of resources, knowledge of health insurance and funding sources, client activation, empowerment and engagement, and the ability to effect change and perform ongoing evaluation.

Professional case managers are licensed and qualified health care professionals (e.g., registered nurses, social workers, and other interdisciplinary team members) who help provide an array of services to assist consumers and their families. Professional case managers help consumers cope with complicated health or medical situations in the most effective way possible, thereby achieving a better quality of life. They help people identify their goals, needs, and resources. From that assessment, the professional case manager and the consumer—whether an individual or a family—together formulate a plan to meet those goals. The professional case manager helps consumers to find resources and facilitates connection with those services. The professional case manager may advocate on behalf of a consumer to obtain needed services. The professional case manager also maintains communication with the consumer to evaluate whether the plan is effective in meeting the consumer's goals. Professional case managers must meet the qualifications outlined in Section III of the CM Model Act of 2017.

Professional Case Manager Qualifications

Professional case managers shall maintain competence in their area(s) of practice by having one of the following: (a) current, active, and unrestricted licensure or certification in a health or human services discipline that allows the professional to conduct an assessment independently as permitted within the scope of practice of the discipline; and/or (b) baccalaureate or graduate degree in social work, nursing, or another health or human services field that promotes the physical, psychosocial, and/or vocational well-being of the persons being served. The degree must be from an institution that is fully accredited by a nationally recognized educational accreditation organization; and the individual must have completed a supervised field experience in case management, health, or behavioral health, as part of the degree requirements.

The professional case manager is one who has the license/certification to conduct an independent assessment, can use critical thinking skills, has the knowledge to develop an individualized plan of care, and can see that it is successfully implemented, impacting quality and safety. Specific professional case manager qualifications will be selected depending on the focus and scope of the case management services being established in the proposed legislation.

Case Management Process

Primary steps in the case management process shall include consumer identification, selection, and engagement in professional case management:

- Establish and implement criteria for identifying individuals for case management services.
- Identify and select consumers who can most benefit from case management services available in a particular practice setting.

- Focus on screening consumers identified or referred by other professionals for case management to determine appropriateness for, and benefits from, services.
- Engage the consumer and family or family caregiver in the process.
- Obtain consent for case management services as part of the case initiation process.

Assessment and opportunity identification:

- Assessment begins after screening, identification, and engagement in case management. It involves data gathering, analysis, and synthesis of information for the purpose of developing a consumer-centered case management plan of care.
- Assessment helps establish the consumer–professional case manager's relationship and the consumer's readiness to engage in his or her own health and well-being. It requires the use of effective communication skills such as active listening, meaningful conversation, motivational interviewing, and use of open-ended questions.
- Care needs and opportunities are identified through analysis of the assessment findings and determination of identified needs, barriers, and/or gaps in care.
- Assessment is an ongoing process occurring intermittently, as needed, to determine efficacy of the case management plan of care and the consumer's progress toward achieving target goals.
- Assessment should cover medical, behavioral health, substance use and abuse, and social determinants of health.
- The professional case manager shall complete a comprehensive, culturally, and linguistically appropriate assessment of each consumer.

Development of the case management plan of care:

- The case management plan of care is a structured, dynamic tool used to document the opportunities, interventions, and expected goals the professional case manager applies during the consumer's engagement in case management services. It includes identified care needs, barriers and opportunities for collaboration with the consumer, family and/or family caregiver, and members of the interprofessional care team to provide more effective integrated care, prioritized goals and/or outcomes to be achieved, and interventions or actions needed to reach the goals.

- Consumer and/or consumer's family or family caregiver input and participation in the development of the case management plan of care are essential to
  - promote consumer-centered care and maximize potential for achieving the target goals;
  - maximize the consumer's health, wellness, safety, adaptation, and self-care;
  - implement policies to promote the autonomy of the consumer, and support the consumer and family decision making; the case management plan of care is put into action by facilitating the coordination of care, services, resources, and health education specified in the planned interventions; effective care coordination requires ongoing communication and collaboration with the consumer and/or consumer's family or family caregiver, as well as the provider and the entire interprofessional health care team;
  - support the physician or practitioner/consumer relationship and plan of care;
  - emphasize prevention of exacerbations and complications utilizing EBP guidelines and consumer empowerment strategies (AHRQ, 2016).

REFERENCES

Agency for Healthcare Research and Quality. (2016). Care Coordination. Retrieved from https://www.ahrq.gov/professionals/prevention -chronic-care/improve/coordination/index.html

American Speech-Language-Hearing Association. (n.d.). Evidence-based practice (EBP). Retrieved from http://www.asha.org/Research/EBP

Boshier, M. (2011, July/August). CCMC News and Views: Understanding new order for care delivery. *Professional Case Management, 16*(4), 168–169. doi:10.1097/NCM.0b013e31821dba53

Case Management Society of America. (2016). *Standards of practice for case management*. Little Rock, AR: Author. Retrieved from http://solutions .cmsa.org/acton/media/10442/standards-of-practice-for-case-management

Newman, M. B. (2017, June). Keeping the "professional" in professional case management. *CMSA Today*. Retrieved from https://www.cmsatoday .com/2016/06/03/keeping-the-professional-in-professional-case-management

Powell, S. K. (2008). How case managers impact patient lives and healthcare dollars. *Professional Case Management, 13*(2), 57–58. doi:10.1097/01 .PCAMA.0000314172.71166.47

Mechanics of Integrated Case Management, Health Complexity, and Integration Between Behavioral Health and Physical Health

Rebecca Perez

Kathleen Fraser

The white man talks about the mind and body and spirit as if they are separate. For us they are one. Our whole life is spiritual, from the time we get up until we go to bed.

—Yakima healer

OBJECTIVES

- Definition of health complexity
- Literature support
- Identification of medically complex populations
- Definition of the ICM process
- Qualifications and training
- Clinical versus nonclinical roles
- Issues and requirements of mental health parity and its impact on case management

Working with complex patients may be one of the greatest challenges case managers face. Complex patients require multidimensional assistance in order to reduce complexity. The historical biomedical approach is ineffective in helping complex patients regain stability; the focus has been on diseases and conditions. The integrated case management model teaches us to focus on the person challenged with medical, behavioral, and social issues to systematically help an individual regain health and function.

Health complexity is a multifaceted description of the challenges an individual may experience and there may be multiple interpretations or definitions accepted by those in health care. Health complexity may include the presence of both medical and behavioral conditions, multiple chronic illnesses, the presence of social concerns, poor access to needed care and services, impairments or disabilities, and financial concerns. Health complexity is often measured by the severity of an illness or level of care acuity. All components of complexity contribute to and impact the measurement of risk an individual may experience. For example, an individual with hypertension would not be considered "complex," but if that same individual has early dementia and forgets to take the prescribed medication, risk is present; or if the individual cannot afford the out-of-pocket expense related to the prescribed medication, adherence to treatment is threatened and therefore risk is present.

Primary care physicians (PCPs) care for individuals with multiple medical conditions and likely spend the majority of their practice hours with these patients. As mentioned, there may be many interpretations of complexity but researchers from Colorado categorized complexity in their article "Primary Care Physician Insights Into a Typology of the Complex Patient in Primary Care" into four categories (Loeb, Binswanger, Candrian, & Bayliss, 2015):

- Medical complexity
  - Includes discordant conditions, chronic pain, medication intolerance, unexplained symptoms, and cognitive issues
- Socioeconomic factors
  - Unaffordability of medications, family stressors, and low levels of health literacy
- Mental illness
  - Depression that results in poor medication adherence, addiction, and anxiety

- Behaviors and traits
  - Demanding, argumentative, and anxiousness

The research conducted by the authors was important to better understand how PCPs conceptualize complexity to improve patient care. One-on-one interviews were conducted with internal medicine physicians who discussed patients they identified as complex. It is important to note that the physicians interviewed differentiated complex patients from "difficult" patients. Difficult patients are those who have challenging personalities but are not necessarily medically complex. Some of the physicians shared specific challenges related to working with the complex patient. Mental illness was identified as a barrier to treating medical illness; for example, depression specifically was identified as a condition that does not always respond to treatment. The experience of hopelessness that may be experienced with depression affects treatment adherence. Homelessness presents challenges because the physician is unable to locate and follow the patient's progress. Another challenge mentioned was abuse and the patient's choice not to leave the abusive environment.

Patients with a higher level of complexity obviously require more intensive support and resources. The primary author of this research hopes to better define medical complexity so that patients are identified earlier so that more intensive interventions can be implemented. This research defined complexity based on interviews with physicians caring for patients with multiple medical, mental, and social conditions. Perhaps complexity cannot be easily defined, or does not quite follow a set of guidelines. Perhaps complexity may be defined as any situation that does not fit a particular set of guidelines or algorithm.

The Case Management Society of America's (CMSA) Integrated Case Management Program has and continues to focus on the following categories and their interaction:

1. Physical health (biological)
2. Behavioral health (psychological)
3. Social
4. Health system

While similar to the research included here, the CMSA categories are based more on the case manager's world view: the patient's challenges and opportunities and how best to assist the patient.

Individuals with complex medical conditions are typically a small percentage of a population but are responsible for using the majority of health care resources. Case management is a strategy implemented to improve access to care and quality of life while reducing the use of health care resources. An estimated 5% of the population uses 50% of health care resources (Goodell, Bodenheimer, & Berry-Miller, 2009). Individuals with five or more chronic conditions spend five times more for health care than those with no chronic conditions (Figure 2.1; Goodell et al., 2009).

How are patients identified for case management? Identifying and stratifying patients most likely to benefit from care management intervention is our target. Case management is a relatively intensive and costly service. Offering case management to patients who are not expected to be high utilizers of hospital, specialty, and emergency department (ED) care would not reduce costs. Similarly, case management for patients too sick to benefit is ineffective.

The health care reform policies implemented in recent years focused on efforts to improve quality and efficiency within health care systems. However, we see significant variation in quality across conditions and settings. To truly improve quality and efficiency, those at the highest risk for poor quality outcomes and significant costs require a special

FIGURE 2.1 Average per capita spending by number of chronic conditions.

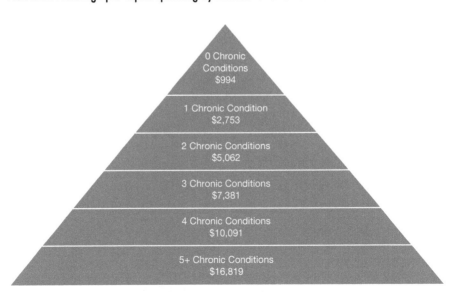

Source: From Goodell et al. (2009).

focus. CMSA's Integrated Case Management approach can be that specific focus.

The 5% of the population mentioned earlier are those with comorbid medical and behavioral conditions. Fragmentation in care and lack of awareness of the need to link medical and mental conditions have resulted in higher health care costs and lack of quality in the care received. These problems are of more concern and burden than the conditions themselves. Evidence-based treatment is available for nearly every disease or condition but implementation is inconsistent.

Medical conditions are more easily diagnosed than behavioral disorders. Behavioral/mental conditions cannot be diagnosed with traditional testing like blood tests, x-rays, and scans. There is no HgA1c to diagnose a mental illness. Mental conditions are typically diagnosed by patient self-report, health utilization data (claims for ED use and admissions and other outpatient access in the medical system), symptoms observed and reported, clinical interviews, and criteria-based scales.

A review of resource utilization will capture those with a mental health diagnosis. Reported symptoms and clinical interventions capture those who meet criteria for a mental disorder regardless of receiving a diagnosis or treatment. Of concern is that less than one-third of individuals meeting criteria for a mental disorder will actually receive condition-changing treatment. The prevalence of mental disorders must also be taken into account in the lifetime experiences of the individual.

The presence of comorbidities between mental and medical conditions is more common than not. Benjamin Druss and Elizabeth Reisinger Walker report that more than 80% of individuals with a mental health condition diagnosed by clinical interview also have at least one general medical condition, and 29% of individuals with a medical condition have mental health comorbidities (2011). They add:

- Individuals with diabetes are two times more likely to have depression versus those without diabetes.

- Individuals with asthma are two to three times more likely to have depression than those without asthma.

- Individuals with cardiovascular disease are 1.43 times more likely to have anxiety.

With every chronic medical condition, the likelihood of developing a comorbid depressive disorder diagnosed by a screening tool increases.

FIGURE 2.2 Percentages of U.S. adults with medical conditions and/or mental disorders.

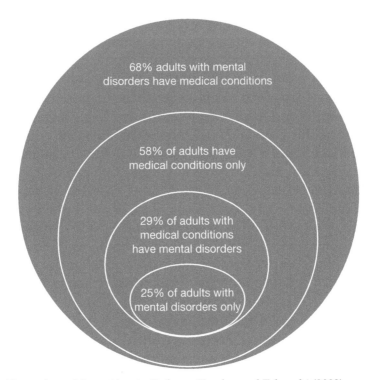

Source: Data adapted from Alegria, Jackson, Kessler, and Takeuchi (2003).

Based on the 1999 National Health Interview Survey, Druss and Walker continue:

- There is a 5% prevalence of depression when no chronic medical condition is present.
- There is a 10% prevalence of depression when two chronic medical conditions are present.
- There is a 12% prevalence of depression when three medical conditions are present. (2011)

Individuals with bipolar disorder or schizophrenia are three times more likely to have three or more chronic conditions. According to the RWJ Synthesis Report titled, "Mental Disorders and Medical Comorbidities," "Medical disorders may lead to mental disorders, mental disorders may place a person at risk for mental disorders, and mental and medical disorders may share common risk factors." When medical conditions present with high symptom burden, depression is common. Examples include chronic back pain and migraines. By the same token, major depression can contribute to the development of medical conditions like cardiovascular disease (2011).

The Integrated Case Management Process

The integrated case management (ICM) process follows CMSA's Standards of Practice for guidance and accountability in case management practice, and is designed to impact individuals with health complexity by a single point of contact, or primary case manager. Just as with any patient, the assessment identifies the patient's needs in four primary domains: biological (medical), psychological (behavioral/mental), social, and health system. However, what should be the priority is the development of a trusting relationship with the patient. We are asking the patient to share with us intimate details of life. The patient must feel that he or she can trust us and believe we genuinely demonstrate empathy and concern for his or her well-being.

To begin working with patients in this manner, our approach should not be robotic or indifferent. The integrated case manager should begin a conversation that establishes who we are and our purpose for contact. The relationship between patients and case manager should be one of advocacy and support. Rather than jumping right in and interrogating patients about their diabetes or asthma, start the encounter by asking what is most important to them, what are their concerns, what worries do they have, what do they need help with; even asking, "So, how can I best help you?"

Individuals with health complexity typically have a long history of health and social challenges. Their experiences with the health care system may be less than satisfactory. Gaining patients' trust is the only way they will be willing to share the intimate details of their lives and health.

An integrated assessment investigates history, current state, and future risk. History cannot be changed but may be a predictor of future risk. In the biological, social, and health system domains, we concern ourselves only with the past 6 months—what conditions and symptoms have been present during this time. An appendectomy or admission for pneumonia greater than 5 years ago really has no impact on the patient's current health; however, the presence of hypertension or diabetes will. These are conditions that regardless of when they were diagnosed are biological challenges. From the social perspective, we look at past disruptions in relationships, work history, residential stability, and presence of support. The last 6 months of health system history include a patient's access to care and relationships with providers. For the patient's status, we assess his or her ability and choices in access to care. The psychological domain is the exception. We look at the lifetime presence of any behavioral conditions as these do have an impact on status as well as future risk. The current status examines the presence of any mental or behavioral symptoms and any barriers that may prevent adherence to treatment.

The status of all four domains reviews symptoms and experiences in the last 30 days. Future risk for all domains requires the case manager to examine history and status to determine the level of risk the patient may experience over the next 3 to 6 months. The result of this comprehensive assessment assists the case manager and the patient in making decisions about where the greatest risk lies and where to begin working to mitigate that risk. This is where the process of care planning begins. The patient's preferences and goals need to be considered the priority, unless of course the patient is at some significant life risk. Prioritizing goals and ability and willingness to implement actions to achieve those goals need to be discussed and negotiated with the patient.

The CMSA's Integrated Case Management model uses an assessment tool, the ICM-CAG (Integrated Case Management Complexity Assessment Grid) which assists the case manager and patient in prioritizing risk. The tool walks us through the four domains, history, status using a scoring, and methodology that will define the risk. The risk scores are color coded making it very easy to identify the highest level of risk and areas of greatest concern.

Green: no risk

Yellow: requires monitoring

Orange: attention required

Red: immediate risk

Individuals with health complexities may have multiple needs. The results of the comprehensive assessment may reveal many areas of risk. Addressing all of the immediate risks at one time may be overwhelming not only to the case manager but also to the patient. Prioritization of the immediate risks using good clinical judgment is required to develop a care plan that will result in success for the patient and the case manager. The presence of multiple risks may also require that the care plan and work with the patient be conducted in incremental steps. For example, a patient with uncontrolled diabetes, chronic obstructive pulmonary disease (COPD), and living in an abusive environment is at multiple risks. So, where to start? We cannot expect this patient to take medications, follow a diet, quit smoking, and move from the abuse all at one time. So, what needs to happen first? This is discussed and negotiated with the patient: "What do you think needs to happen first?" Likely helping the patient feel safe would be the primary concern; assisting the patient find a safe place to live will hopefully reduce fear, anxiety, and stress allowing for more of a focus on health. The full ICM process will be discussed in detail using case studies later in the manual.

Qualifications and Training

Case managers are licensed health care professionals or those who hold advanced degrees in health and human services. Experienced case managers are familiar with the processes related to assessment, care planning, advocacy, facilitation, and care coordination. Traditionally, case managers practice within the discipline with which they are most familiar or for which their clinical practice was focused. For example, a medical case manager with a strong background in maternal/child health works with women who have high-risk pregnancies. But if the pregnant patient is currently using heroin, the medical case manager will refer the patient to a behavioral health case manager to address the patient's addiction. This means that two case managers are outreaching the patient instead of one single point of contact with whom the patient can develop a trusting relationship. Coincidentally, a behavioral health case manager is working with a patient who has had multiple admissions for psychotic breaks. The patient has not been taking medications as prescribed to manage schizophrenia. The lack of schizophrenic symptom management has also resulted in the patient developing a wound from uncontrolled diabetes. Typically, the issue of uncontrolled diabetes and the wound would be addressed by a medical case manager; again, no single point of contact for the patient.

The ICM model requires case managers, regardless of background, to address all conditions and needs of a patient. Many case managers feel uncomfortable addressing conditions with which they are unfamiliar or do not routinely address. First and foremost, case managers must understand that they do not diagnose and do not treat. While it is understandable that a case manager may feel less than confident in addressing a less familiar condition, it is expected when practicing an integrated approach that the case manager take the initiative to understand all the patient's conditions. This is part of the case manager's professional growth and stewardship required to be an effective advocate and support. Learning about conditions is not the only strategy for being better prepared to support your patients. Consultations with peers who may have experience in the area where you do not can be most valuable. Your peers can share their experiences to help you better understand the patient's conditions and suggest strategies that have worked. Consulting with medical directors will also result in guidance.

According to the RWJ Foundation Synthesis Project, the literature was reviewed to evaluate the effectiveness of case/care management; the key to successful case management programs and interventions include (Goodell et al., 2009):

- In-person encounters
  - Home visits
- Training and personnel
  - Specially trained case managers
  - Low workloads
  - Registered nurses (RNs) working as part of an interdisciplinary team
- Physician involvement
  - Case managers in the primary care setting are especially effective in facilitating collaboration with physicians
  - Case managers from payor organizations embedded in practices and clinics can achieve the same as case managers employed by the physician practice

- Informed caregivers
  - Includes family, long-term care providers, community health workers
  - Essential to assist with observation and reporting functional and cognitive decline
  - Collaborative support between caregivers and case managers
- Coaching
  - Teaching patients and caregivers how to recognize early warning signs of complications and worsening conditions
  - Provide strategies to promote management of conditions

Case managers assist patients and their support system in managing both behavioral and medical conditions through care coordination, support, advocacy, and mitigation of barriers. To function as integrated case managers, we need to be licensed health care professionals or have an advanced degree in a health and human services discipline. Ideally, case managers with experience will be better prepared for the challenges of multidimensional support of complex patients. Experience is an asset but additional training is also needed. Training should include:

- Motivational interviewing training to assist with decisions to make change
- Cross-disciplinary training in medical and behavioral conditions and an understanding of how conditions interact to cause complexity
- Relationship development for improved patient engagement

Clinical Versus Nonclinical Roles

Not every member of a health population will require case management. As discussed earlier, only a small percentage of a population will experience complexity. However, some others may need some level of health or social support from nonclinical care coordinators, health coaching, or short-term case management. In this manual, we are focusing on the most complex individuals of a population.

The RWJ Synthesis Report for Care Management for Patients with Complex Health Needs supports the recommendation we make that a case manager should function as part of a multidisciplinary team to support care and services for the complex patient (Goodell et al., 2009). Of added importance to remember, the triage process is essential to ensuring the complex patient is assigned the most appropriate primary case manager. This triage process should be based on the patient's risk. Where does the greatest risk lie? In the behavioral domain or the medical domain? The primary diagnosis that is causing the greatest risk should guide the assignment of the primary case manager.

CASE STUDY 1

Julia is a 44-year-old with uncontrolled diabetes, daily blood sugars fluctuating between 50 before breakfast and 300 after dinner, a non-healing wound on her left foot, and chronic depression.

Should the primary case manager have a medical background or a behavioral background?

The greatest risk lies with the patient's uncontrolled blood sugars. Severe fluctuations in blood sugar put the patient at risk of admission and worsening of the wound. However, the patient's depression is likely contributing to her poor control. The case manager must work with the patient to discover how best to address her depression so that she can focus on diabetes management. ∎ ∎ ∎

CASE STUDY 2

Roger has been admitted for heroin overdose three times in the last 6 months. He also has been diagnosed with COPD and has been to the ED for shortness of breath four times in the last year because he continues to smoke and does not use the long-acting inhaler prescribed by his PCP.

Should the primary case manager have a medical background or a behavioral background?

The greatest risk lies with a potential for death. Roger has already had three heroin overdoses in the last 6 months. If his substance abuse is not addressed, the next overdose could be fatal, so his primary case manager should be a behavioral health case manager. Addressing his smoking and medication nonadherence is important but unless he stops heroin use, it is unlikely the COPD exacerbations will be controlled. ▪ ▪ ▪

Cases such as these support the need for good triage practices that include critical thinking to make good clinical decisions. The primary case managers should also be supported by an interdisciplinary team. Case managers working with complex populations may be assigned very small caseloads as these patients take more time to engage and follow. They have high needs across the domains and if the primary case manager is to meet all the patient's needs, a significant amount of time is required. The ICM model recommends that case care teams be developed within the case management organization or place of practice. The care team is made up of both clinical and nonclinical staff. The nonclinical staff can assist the primary case manager's coordination of services like scheduling provider appointments, handling correspondence, and arranging for delivery of durable medical equipment (DME) or medical supplies. These tasks do not necessarily require patient contact but are essential for care coordination. In order to ensure effective use of resources, medical and behavioral case managers should spend their time working with clients and patients.

A suggested care team includes:

Medical case managers

Behavioral case managers

Nonclinical support staff or case management extenders

Community health workers

Pharmacy staff

Medical directors

Health coaches

The medical and behavioral case managers support each other with their respective experiences. The nonclinical staff assists with coordination activities that do not require clinical expertise. Pharmacy staff assist with medication review and reconciliation. Community health workers can be the eyes and ears of the case manager if telephonic and can become peer supports for the patients. Medical directors guide the case managers by advising on best practice, evidence-based practice, and can be a liaison with providers. The members of the care team support each other while taking ownership of the patients they serve.

Mental Health Parity and Integrated Case Management

Historically, individuals with mental health conditions have been viewed as difficult to treat. Under the Affordable Care Act (ACA) passed in 2010, behavioral health services were included as one of the 10 essential benefits, meaning that insurers were required to cover mental health services equally to that of medical services.

In the United States, one in four Americans will experience a mental health condition each year, and approximately 50% of Americans will develop a mental disorder in their lifetimes while 28% will develop an addiction (Boerner, 2014). Individuals with behavioral issues and/or addictions visit the ED more frequently, are more likely to be admitted, and have a higher rate of readmission (2014). Nearly 80% of individuals admitted to the hospital have comorbid psychiatric disorders (2014). These disorders make management of physical conditions like diabetes, hypertension, or heart disease difficult and have poor outcomes. The ACA established an expectation that physicians would coordinate both physical and mental health services and treatment. There is evidence that demonstrates integration of care could save money and improve outcomes (2014).

The shortage of behavioral health providers significantly challenges the ability to coordinate behavioral and medical services. In large accountable care organizations (ACO), it is much easier as the disciplines are co-located. This is common in urban areas. The co-location of both medical and behavioral health professionals in clinics and primary care practices allows the patient to address all his or her needs in one visit rather than seeing multiple providers in multiple locations. An early study of collaborative care demonstrated a 42% drop in ED visits when primary care was offered in a behavioral health clinic (Boerner, 2014). In a Florida program, inpatient admissions were reduced from 17% to 10% when outpatient psychiatric care was better coordinated (2014).

For providers who are not integrated, it is much more difficult to demonstrate these kinds of outcomes because there are not enough behavioral specialists available. The National Alliance for Mental Illness (NAMI) reported in 2011 that more than half of all U.S. counties lacked even one psychiatrist, psychologist, or social worker (Boerner, 2014). The ACA provides coverage for behavioral health services but in many cases access to providers is limited or very limited. Another concern is reimbursement because many insurers have traditionally contracted out behavioral services and employers have independently contracted with separate companies for these services. Mental health utilization practices may be stringent and coordination and collaboration with the medical sector are absent. These types of contractual arrangements threaten the ability to integrate care. Mental health specialist groups and independent companies are not working with primary care and usually document in a different documentation system or health record. Individual case managers are challenged with helping many patients access needed behavioral services timely and within close geographic proximity. Attempts to integrate care may become the responsibility of the case manager to facilitate and coordinate care between providers.

REFERENCES

Alegria, M., Jackson J. S., Kessler, R. C., & Takeuchi, D. (2003). National Comorbidity Survey Replication (NCS-R), 2001–2003. Ann Arbor, MI: Inter-university Consortium for Political and Social Research.

Druss, B. G., & Walker, E. R. (2011). *Mental disorders and medical comorbidity* (Research synthesis report no. 21). Princeton, NJ: The Robert Wood Johnson Foundation. Retrieved from https://www.rwjf .org/content/dam/farm/reports/issue_briefs/2011/rwjf69438/ subassets/rwjf69438_1

Boerner, H. (2014). Mental health parity: Where it has been and where it's going. *Physician Executive Journal, 40,* 74–76. Retrieved from https://slideblast.com/queue/mental-health-parity-where-it-has-been-and-where-its-_5981b6b11723ddf3a1d1c991.html

Goodell, S., Bodenheimer, T., & Berry-Miller, R. (2009). *The Synthesis Project: Care management of patients with complex health care needs* (Policy brief no. 19). Princeton, NJ: The Robert Wood Johnson Foundation. ISSN: 2155-3718

Loeb, D. F., Binswanger, I. A., Candrian, C., & Bayliss, E. A. (2015). Primary care physician insights into a typology of the complex patient in primary care. *The Annals of Family Medicine, 13,* 451–455. doi:10.1370/afm.1840

CHAPTER 3

Global Models of Integrated Case Management

Corine Latour

For clinical use, be open as a provider to look at an new way of assessing medical complexity, it benefits multidisciplinary work.

—2017 INTERMED Consortium

OBJECTIVES

- Understand the concept, roles, and functions of the INTERMED program
- Understand the case analysis and review of research from each project and specific patient populations (e.g., frail elderly, workers' compensation)
- Summarize key issues with the INTERMED self-assessment pilot
- Understand the key organizational and case management needs related to the INTERMED process
- Understand the issues and requirements of Mental Health Parity and the impact of integrated case management

In Western countries, health care workers, policy makers, and politicians are seeking ways to (a) improve population health, (b) improve care, and (c) reduce costs per capita. This so-called triple aim principle was developed by Berwick, Nolan, and Whittington (2008). It sequels the previously published report *Crossing the Quality Chasm* from 2001 (Institute of Medicine Committee on Quality Health Care in America, 2001) whereby effective, safe, timely, appropriate, patient-centered, and accessible care for all was mentioned.

After the publication by Berwick, Bisognano and Kenney (2012) published the book *Pursuing the Triple Aim*. They describe seven innovative improvements in health care. Although these initiatives are innovative, it is notable that they do not often take into account that a number of our patients have comorbidities, often psychiatric and somatic diseases, often have a poor social system, low economic status, and not to forget do not have a very high trust in health care and health care workers.

Health care in Europe as well as in the United States includes a number of organizing principles. To begin with, there is the dichotomy between somatic and mental health care. Next, there is the point of determining whether or not the problem is urgent. Then there are the specializations, which have become increasingly divided into sub-specializations where consulting hours are sometimes tailored to one diagnosis only, for instance at a diabetes clinic or a multiple sclerosis (MS) consultation. And then there are the insurance requirements, which strictly define what can and cannot be claimed.

From a strictly medical and financial point of view, this approach may be rational, but many patients do not fit into such a system because they suffer from combinations of diseases or do not behave like "standard patients." Every social worker and nurse know that some patients can require much more time and energy than other patients, even though they all come in with the same medical problem. For those time- and energy-consuming patients, case management is needed. The challenge we are facing is how to timely identify those so-called complex patients.

In general, patients with a chronic disease, in Europe and in the United States, have access to a treatment team consisting of a variety of disciplines. For example, patients with diabetes have access to a treatment team consisting of an internist, a dietician, a podiatrist, an ophthalmologist, a neurologist, a specialist diabetes nurse, and a social worker. We call this a "disease management team": a team that can effectively cope with the complications that can occur in such a chronic disease. These teams are set up according to the "chronic care model" (Wagner, 2000) in which the team provides multidisciplinary preventive long-term care and encourages patients to actively participate in their care. The treatment outcome is determined largely by the degree to which the patient is able to meet the requirements associated with the treatment. It is easy to imagine that if someone is suffering from depression or the early stages of dementia in addition to diabetes, this will have a negative impact on the degree of cooperation from, and collaboration with, the patient. For these patients, a more integrated and biopsychosocial approach is appropriate. Such an approach focuses less on the causes of the problems, and more on the connections between them (Leentjes, Gans, Schols, & van Weel, 2010). This sort of integrated approach is suitable for patient groups such as:

- The frail elderly
- Patients with chronic physical illnesses who suffer from concomitant psychiatric disorders such as anxiety disorders, depression, or addiction
- Patients who develop cognitive disorders as a result of physical illnesses, such as dementia with Parkinson's disease or mood disorders with multiple sclerosis
- Patients who develop physical illnesses due to their troubled or complex behavior, such as patients who self-harm or patients with severe eating disorders; and last but not least
- Patients who have chronic complaints about their physical state, although no clearly identifiable physical condition can be found (Huyse & Latour, 2009)

Case management is defined by the Case Management Society of America (CMSA) as: "A collaborative process of assessment, planning, facilitation, care coordination, evaluation and advocacy for options and services to facilitate an individual's and family's comprehensive health needs through communication and available resources to promote patient safety, quality of care, and cost effective outcomes" (CMSA, 2016). It is not for nothing that the process of assessment is mentioned first. Without a proper assessment, there is a great risk to give inappropriate care, in an ineffective way which, in the long run, will lead to poor health care, higher costs, and clients who will be less satisfied and less trustful of the health care they received. A case manager is very important for timely identification of so-called complex patients.

Integrated Case Management

As mentioned in the introduction, there is a wide variety in the ways we organize our care in Western countries, but there are similarities in our case loads. Knowing this, it is a utopia to think that there is only one model that fits all. One can be inspired by best practices, bearing in mind that a best practice is not always the best for your practice. An understanding of necessary conditions will help to set up a good practice.

1. Case management should consist of the following core components:
    a. Case finding
    b. Assessment
    c. Care planning
    d. Care coordination (i.e., medication management, self-care support), involving the system (family, friends), psychological support, and so on (Ross, Curry, & Goodwin, 2011)
2. Case management for patients in need of the in-depth tools of the INTERMED is most effective when performed only for our most complex patients.
3. The case manager needs to be embedded in a wider system that supports and values integrated care (Ross et al., 2011).
4. To deliver better care for patients by carrying out a case management program, nurses or case managers should be trained to work as case managers. Case finding (by using the INTERMED or INTERMED self-assessment tool), motivational interviewing techniques, and shared decision making (see Chapter 5) are essential parts of a case manager–training program.

Case Finding and Assessment of "Complex Patients" by the INTERMED Self-Assessment (IM-SA)

As described, health complexity is defined as the interference with standard care by the interaction of biological, psychological, social, and health system factors.

To get a better handle on patient complexity and care complexity, a measurement instrument such as the INTERMED Complexity Assessment Grid (IM-CAG) method can be used to identify complex patients. With this method we can explore how to improve the structure and efficiency of care for this relatively small patient group that generates relatively large costs. The IM-CAG method was developed in order to identify patients with complex care needs and provide them with the proper care (van

Reedt Dortland et al., 2017). It is based on the biopsychosocial or integrated approach. The IM-CAG method allows one to analyze the complexity of adult and elderly patients in all types of care facilities, including hospitals, outpatient clinics, and other local care settings. The connection between the risk-weighting and corresponding-action levels qualifies the IM method as a decision analysis method. By means of an interview, the care provider gathers information about the patient's physical (biological), mental, and social state, as well as details on the care provided, in order to gain a better understanding of the risks involved in caring for this patient. After having been identified in the interview, the risks are weighted.

This risk-weighting process simultaneously yields an indication of what should be done with these risks: nothing (green), monitor (yellow), intervene (orange), or take drastic and immediate action (red). Because the risks are arranged in a diagram and their weighting is indicated by colors, an overview is provided in a single figure. This overview can be used to facilitate coordination between disciplines, which is essential when dealing with complex patients.

A disadvantage of the IM-CAG interview is that it is time consuming. An interview will take approximately 20 minutes and the elaboration of the answers another 20 minutes. For that the INTERMED consortium developed the IM-Self Assessment (IM-SA, 2015) questionnaire as an alternative for the IM-CAG. A validity study was carried out whereby 850 patients (ages 17–90) from five different countries in Europe completed the IM-SA and were evaluated with the IM. The research group concluded that "the IM-SA is a generic and time-efficient method to assess biopsychosocial complexity and to provide guidance for multidisciplinary care trajectories in adult patients, with good reliability and validity across different cultures" (van Reedt Dortland et al., 2017). Complementary to the INTERMED-Elderly-Self-Assessment (IM-E-SA) has been developed. The IM-E-SA has, in contrast to the IM-SA, no questions related to occupational activities and has an extra item on whether patients live by the day and do not think about possible changes (in prognosis) in the future. The reliability and validity of the IM-E-SA were good (Peters et al., 2015).

Notable is that the patients, in general, filling out the IM-SA, estimate their own situation as less complex than health care workers do when they interview the patient. Although the validity of the IM-SA was proved, one should always bear in mind that a self-assessment questionnaire differs from a semi-structured interview by a case manager:

TABLE 3.1 IM-CAG Versus IM-SA, Two Different Worlds

IM-CAG	IM-SA
Professional interview	Person
Normative interpretation	Narrative interpretation
Evidence	Emotions
Uniformity	Creativity
Protocols	Diversity

IM-CAG, INTERMED-Complexity Assessment Grid; IM-SA, INTERMED-Self Assessment.

To understand the meaning of the differences detailed in Table 3.1, it is important to understand the meaning of "etic" and "emic":

"Etic" represents the perspective from the outside. How does an outsider (for instance the case manager) see a particular reality?

"Emic" represents the perspective from the inside, how someone experiences him- or herself. What is the meaning for the patient, and how does he or she imagine and explain things (Kottak, 2006)?

It is understandable that a case manager values and interprets the situation of a patient differently than a patient does:

CASE STUDY 1

At your consultation hour, you see Ms. Lennard, mother of two young children, suffering from diabetes and having a drug addiction. She is unemployed. The father of the children, her ex-husband, takes care of the rent of her house. You interview the patient (IM-CAG) and your first idea is that the diabetes and the drug addiction should be treated, despite the fact that several health care workers were not very successful in motivating the patient for treatment. You have no worries about the living circumstances since there are no debts and the ex-husband pays the rent. You ask the patient to fill out an IM-self assessment questionnaire and, to your surprise, she filled out that an immediate adjustment for the living situation is needed. When you discuss this with the patient, she reasons as follows: she lives in a neighborhood where drug dealers live and work and she realizes that as long as she lives in this area, she will not be able to stop the use of hard drugs. But to move to another area, she needs to have a job, because the rent in the "better areas" is higher; for that she needs to stop using drugs and engage in healthier habits in order to keep her diabetes under control.

Thus, although the patient and the case manager end up with the same conclusion: treatment of the diabetes and drug addiction, the "route of thinking" to come to this conclusion was different. The case manager followed the reasoning of the patient, using motivational interviewing and shared decision-making techniques. ■ ■ ■

For this it is good to realize that the way we perform as case managers is usually from a perspective of *needs* of a patient instead of *wishes* or *desires* of the patient. To discuss the outcome of the IM-SA you will get a better understanding of the perspective of the patient.

CASE STUDY 2

The family doctor asked you, the case manager, to visit Mr. Hussein, 87 years old, living alone in a small but comfortable house with his five cats. Mr. Hussein is very much on his own; he was never married and has no children. He worked very hard his whole life; there are no financial problems. The family doctor tells you that Mr. Hussein has more and more problems in taking good care of himself. Cooking, doing the laundry, taking care of the house and the garden, it is all too much for him. He visits the doctor regularly with vague physical complaints. You interview him via the IM-CAG method and discuss with him his needs (extra home care, meal delivery, etc.). Mr. Hussein becomes agitated; he wants only to be left alone. You decided to let him fill out an IM-SA. You noticed then that Mr. Hussein is much more positive about his prognoses than you are. You decide to discuss this in an open and unprejudiced way and ask him what his desires and wishes for the future are. He tells you that he is worried about his cats when he is dead. He also tells you that he loves opera and that he really would love to go to the opera house, but can't go on his own. You tell him about the church three blocks from his house that is helping people like him to fulfill wishes such as his. You tell him that the church also organizes dinners three times per week, so maybe he can sign in and see if they can mean anything for him. When talking further,

Mr. Hussein tells you that although he is always very much by himself, it becomes much harder since he's getting older. He asks you to respect the fact that his house is not very clean, as well as his clothes, but he wants you to help him with his wishes. You decide to do so and set up the contact with the church. The nurse-assistant visits Mr. Hussein on a 6-week basis. ■ ■ ■

The INTERMED Self-Assessment

The IM-SA questionnaire contains twenty so-called clinical anchor points; the names of these clinical anchor points are mentioned above the questions. The IM-SA is divided into the same subdomains as in the IM-CAG: Biological, Psychological, Social, and Health System. Each domain is divided into three time segments: History, Current State, and Vulnerability/Prognosis.

The IM-SA consists of the following questions (IM-SA, 2017):

Historical—Biological chronicity

1a. Did you experience any physical problem in the past 5 years?

1b. Do you suffer from one or more long-lasting or chronic diseases (e.g., diabetes, high blood pressure, rheumatoid arthritis, lung disease, or cancer)?

Historical—Diagnostic dilemma

2. How difficult has it been in the past 5 years to diagnose the physical problems you experienced?

Current—Symptom severity

3. How much were your daily activities (e.g., job, house-keeping, hobbies, going out) restricted by physical problems during the last week?

Current—Diagnostic/therapeutic challenge

4a. Do you think your doctors understand the origin of your current physical problem(s)?

4b. Do you think you are receiving the appropriate treatment for your current physical problem(s)?

Historical—Coping

5. In the past 5 years, how did you cope with stressful, difficult situations?

Historical—Mental health

6. In your past, have you ever had psychological problems, such as being tense, anxious, down/blue, or confused?

Current—Resistance to treatment

7. Do you think it is difficult to follow your health caregivers' recommendations?

Current—Mental health symptoms

8. At present, are you experiencing psychological problems, such as being tense, anxious, down/blue, or confused?

Historical—Job and leisure

9a. Do you have a job?

9b. If you said No, please specify:

9c. Do you have activities in your spare time such as volunteering, courses, sports, clubs . . .?

Historical—Social relationships

10. How do you generally relate to other people?

Current—Residential stability

11. Is your home living situation satisfactory? Or are adjustments needed, such as home modifications, receiving home care, or going to live somewhere else?

Current—Social support

12. Is assistance from your partner, family, colleagues, or friends available for you at any time?

Historical—Access to care

13. Do you experience problems in getting the care you need due to living too far away, or not having any insurance, or not speaking the language very well, or differences in culture?

Historical—Treatment experience

14. How did you experience your contacts with doctors and health care providers in the last 5 years?

Current—Organization of care

15. Who are the health care providers who take care for you at the moment? [multiple answers allowed]

Current—Coordination of care

16. To what extent do your doctors and health care providers work together?

Prognosis—Complications and threat

17. In the next 6 months, do you expect your physical health to change? [Try to make the best estimate]

Prognosis—Mental health threat

18. In the next 6 months, do you expect your psychological well-being to change? [Try to make the best estimate]

Prognosis—Social vulnerability

19. In the next 6 months, do you expect that a change will be needed in the way you are currently living? [Try to make the best estimate]

Prognosis—Health system impediments

20. In the next 6 months, do you expect that you will be in need of more help and support? [Try to make the best estimate]

All IM-SA items are, similar to the IM-CAG, scored on a four-level rating scale. The rating scores range from 0 to 3 which represent zero evidence for a symptom, disturbance, or health care need (0) to experienced complex symptoms or health care needs (3). The item markers are comparable with the colors of signal lights, marking the extent of necessity or urgency of the need or wish for action and care-taking. Green (0) denotes that no care taking is necessary or there are no wishes of the patient. The more the color resembles red, the more urgent action is required.

General principle

Green   0 = No vulnerability/need

Yellow   1 = Mild vulnerability/need for monitoring or prevention

Orange   2 = Moderate vulnerability/need for treatment or inclusion in treatment plan

Red   3 = Severe vulnerability/need for immediate or intensive treatment

The total maximum score of the IM-SA is 60. The complexity cutoff point for the IM-CAG is 21; the cutoff point of the IM-SA is 19. A score of 19 or higher indicates complexity (van Reedt Dortland et al., 2017).

To determine the complexity of patients per time segment and per domain, the scores of the single questions are added up according to a configuration table, helping you to come to a complexity score.

REFERENCES

Berwick, D. M., Nolan, T. W., & Whittington, J. (2008). The triple aim: Care, health and cost. *Health Affairs, 27*(3), 759–769. doi:10.1377/hlthaff.27.3.759

Bisognano, M., & Kenney, C. (2012). *Pursuing the triple aim. Seven innovators show the way to better care, better health, and lower costs.* San Francisco, CA: Jossey-Bass. ISBN: 9781118205723

Case Management Society of America. (2016). *Standards of practice for case management.* Little Rock, AR: Author. Retrieved from http://solutions.cmsa.org/acton/media/10442/standards-of-practice-for-case-management

Huyse, F. J., & Latour, C. H. M. (2009). *Geïntegreerde zorg voor complexe patiënten met de INTERMED-methodiek: Handleiding HBO-V* [Integrated care for complex patients with the INTERMED methodology: Manual HBO-V]. Amsterdam, The Netherlands: Amsterdam University of Applied Sciences.

Institute of Medicine Committee on Quality Health Care in America (2001). *Crossing the quality chasm: A new health system for the 21st century.* Washington, DC: National Academies Press. ISBN: 9780309072809

INTERMED-Self Assessment. (2015). Questionnaire. Retrieved from http://www.intermedconsortium.com/wp-content/uploads/2015/08/IMSA_englishPDF_coloured.pdf

Kottak, C. (2006). *Mirror for humanity* (5th ed.). New York, NY: McGraw-Hill. ISBN: 9780073258942

Leentjes, A. F. G., Gans, R. O. B., Schols, J. M. G. A., & van Weel, C. (2010). Integrale geneeskunde: Begripsbepaling, historie en concepten [Integral medicine: Definition of concepts, history and concepts]. In A. F. G. Leentjes, R. O. B. Gans, & J. M. G. A. Schols (Eds.), *Handboek multidisciplinaire zorg [Handbook on multidisciplinary care]* (pp. 9–20). Utrecht, The Netherlands: De Tijdstroom. ISBN: 9789058981745

Peters, L. L., Burgerhof, J. G. M., Boter, H., Wild, B., Buskens, E., & Slaets, J. P. J. (2015). Predictive validity of a frailty measure (GFI) and a case complexity measure (IM-E-SA) on healthcare costs in an elderly population. *Journal of Psychosomatic Research, 79*(5), 404–411. doi:10.1016/j.jpsychores.2015.09.015

Ross, S., Currry, N., & Goodwin, N. (2011). *Case management. What it is and how it can best be implemented.* London, UK: The Kings Fund. ISBN: 9781857176308

van Reedt Dortland, A. K. B., Peters, L. L., Boenink, A. D., Smit, J. H., Slaets, J. P. J., Hoogendoorn, A. W., . . . Ferrari, S. (2017). Assessment of biopsychosocial complexity and health care needs: Measurement properties of the INTERMED self-assessment version. *Psychosomatic Medicine, 79*(4), 485–492. doi:10.1097/PSY.0000000000000446

Wagner, E. H. (2000). The role of patient care teams in chronic disease management. *British Medical Journal, 320,* 569–572. Retrieved from https://www.ncbi.nlm.nih.gov/pmc/articles/PMC1117605/pdf/569.pdf

PART II

Assessment of Patient Populations Using Integrated Case Management

Assessing the Adult Patient Through Application of the Integrated Case Management Complexity Assessment Grid

Rebecca Perez
Kathleen Fraser

Apprehension, uncertainty, waiting, expectation, fear of surprise, do a patient more harm than any exertion.

—Florence Nightingale

OBJECTIVES

- Understand the INTERMED-complexity assessment grid
- Understand the integrated case management–complexity assessment grid
- Understand the point scoring for each complexity item
- Understand the professional case manager's actions with the scores
- Understand nursing documentation related to the Integrated Case Management (ICM) process

This chapter puts into practice the method of integrated case management. We will examine a case study and apply what we learn about the patient to the Integrated Case Management Complexity Assessment Grid (ICM-CAG). The case will be examined in detail looking at the patient's risk and possible actions to consider for a care plan. Examination of each of the risk elements will help you to better understand the application of the ICM-CAG as well as how to systematically address all domains of health.

Basics of the Adult Integrated Case Management Complexity Assessment Grid

The Case Management Society of America's (CMSA's) ICM-CAG was adapted in 2006 from the IM-CAG developed in Europe and was published in *The Integrated Case Management Manual: Assisting Complex Patients Regain Medical and Mental Health* (Kathol, Perez, & Cohen, 2010). CMSA embraced the methodology developed by the INTERMED Foundation (Table 4.1). The ICM-CAG, CMSA's adaptation, is a tool used in conjunction with a comprehensive assessment to systematically demonstrate the presence of strengths and risks. The completion of a comprehensive assessment and use of the ICM-CAG exceed assessment guidelines as outlined in *CMSA's Standards of Practice*. In this chapter, we talk about conducting a comprehensive assessment using the ICM-CAG to guide us in determining levels of health risk. Understanding risk helps us to develop a prioritized plan of care. As scores are applied to the individual risk elements in the ICM-CAG, a final score is applied. Scores greater than 30 indicate complexity, and the higher the score, obviously the greater the complexity. Periodic reassessment using the ICM-CAG can be used as a means of demonstrating outcomes. As we work with a member to reduce risk and improve health, the risk score decreases.

When working with complex patients, an assessment may take more time than anticipated, and should be conducted as a conversation, not as an interrogation. When assessing a patient who experiences a level of complexity, we may need to complete the assessment in more than one encounter, especially if the assessment is conducted telephonically. It is much easier to conduct a comprehensive assessment when meeting the patient face to face. The ICM-CAG helps to demonstrate where the patient's risk(s) lie and provides a score related to that risk. Over time as we work with the patient, we will (hopefully) see the risk score reduced, health improve as well as quality of life.

TABLE 4.1 INTERMED-Complexity Assessment Grid

Date:	HEALTH RISKS AND HEALTH NEEDS						
Name:	HISTORICAL		CURRENT STATE		VULNERABILITY		
Total Score =	Complexity Item	Score	Complexity Item	Score	Complexity Item	Score	
Biological Domain	Chronicity HB1		Symptom Severity/ Impairment CB1		Complications and Life Threat VB		
	Diagnostic Dilemma HB2		Diagnostic Therapeutic Challenge CB2				
Psychological Domain	Barriers to Coping HP1		Resistance to Treatment CP1		Mental Health Threat VP		
	Mental Health History HP2		Mental Health Symptoms CP2				
Social Domain	Job and Leisure HS1		Residential Stability CS1		Social Vulnerability VS		
	Relationships HS2		Social Support CS2				
Health System Domain	Access to Care HHS1		Getting Needed Services CHS1		Health System Impediments VHS		
	Treatment Experience HHS2		Coordination of Care CHS2				

Comments

(Enter pertinent information about the reason for the score of each complexity item here. For example, poor patient adherence, death in family with stress to patient, non-evidence-based treatment of migraine, etc.)

Scoring System
Green   0 = no need to act
Yellow   1 = mild risk and need for monitoring or prevention
Orange   2 = moderate risk and need for action or development of intervention plan
Red   3 = severe risk and need for immediate action or immediate intervention plan

(continued)

TABLE 4.1 INTERMED-Complexity Assessment Grid (*continued*)

Biological Domain Items		Psychological Domain Items	
Chronicity	Physical illness chronicity	Barriers to Coping	Problems handling stress and/or problem solving
Diagnostic Dilemma	Historic problems in the diagnosis of physical illness	Mental Health History	Prior mental condition difficulties
Symptom Severity/ Impairment	Physical illness symptom severity and impairment	Resistance to Treatment	Resistance to treatment; nonadherence
Diagnostic/ Therapeutic Challenge	Current difficulties in current diagnosis and/ or treatment	Mental Health Symptoms	Current mental condition symptom severity
Complications and Life Threat	Risk of physical complications and life threat if case management is stopped	Mental Health Threat	Risk of persistent personal barriers or poor mental condition care if case management is stopped
Social Domain Items		Health System Domain Items	
Job and Leisure	Personal productivity and leisure activities	Access to Care	Health system–related access to appropriate care including reimbursement options for needed services
Relationships	Relationship difficulties	Treatment Experience	Experiences with doctors or the health system
Residential Stability	Residential stability or suitability	Getting Needed Services	Logistical ability to get needed care at service delivery level
Social Support	Availability of social support	Coordination of Care	Communication among providers to ensure coordinated care
Social Vulnerability	Risk of work, home, and relational support needs if case management is stopped	Health System Impediments	Risk of continued poor access to and/or coordination of services if case management is stopped

CB, current biological; CHS, current health system; CP, current psychological; CS, current social; HB, history biological; HHS, history health system; HP, history psychological; HS, history social; VB, vulnerability biological; VHS, vulnerability health system; VP, vulnerability psychological; VS, vulnerability social.

The ICM-CAG has been further developed from that published in the *Integrated Case Management Manual: Assisting Complex Patients Regain Physical and Mental Health* (Kathol, Perez, & Cohen, 2010) to this latest version (Table 4.2), which continues to examine the four domains of

TABLE 4.2 Integrated Case Management-Complexity Assessment Grid

Date:	HEALTH RISKS AND HEALTH NEEDS					
Name:	HISTORICAL		CURRENT STATE		VULNERABILITY	
Total Score =	Complexity Item	Score	Complexity Item	Score	Complexity Item	Score
Biological Domain	Chronic Illness		Symptom Severity/ Impairment		Complications and Life Threat	
	Diagnostic Difficulty		Adherence Ability			
Psychological Domain	Barriers to Coping		Resistance to Treatment		Mental Health Threat	
	Mental Health History		Mental Health Symptoms			
Social Domain	Job and Leisure		Residential Stability		Social Vulnerability	
	Relationships		Social Support			
Health System Domain	Access to Care		Getting Needed Services		Health System Deterrents	
	Treatment Experience		Provider Collaboration			

Comments

(Enter pertinent information about the reason for the score of each complexity item here. For example, poor patient adherence, death in family with stress to patient, non-evidence-based treatment of migraine, etc.)

Scoring System
Green   0 = no need to act
Yellow   1 = mild risk and need for monitoring or prevention
Orange   2 = moderate risk and need for action or development of intervention plan
Red   3 = severe risk and need for immediate action or immediate intervention plan

(continued)

TABLE 4.2 Integrated Case Management-Complexity Assessment Grid (*continued*)

Biological Domain Items		Psychological Domain Items	
Chronic Illness	Physical illness chronicity	Barriers to Coping	Problems handling stress and/or problem solving
Diagnostic Difficulty	Difficulty getting a condition diagnosed; multiple providers consulted; multiple diagnostic tests completed	Mental Health History	Prior mental condition difficulties
Symptom Severity	Physical illness symptom severity and impairment; does the severity of symptoms result in a disability, i.e., unable to care for self, unable to perform ADL or IADL, unable to work or go to school	Resistance to Treatment	Resistance to treatment/non-adherence; doesn't believe the treatment is right for him/her; not following a physician's treatment plan due to poor health literacy/ doesn't understand the goal of treatment; or a behavioral condition has interfered, i.e., depression, anxiety, poorly managed SMI
Adherence Ability	Current difficulties in the ability to follow a physician's treatment plan	Mental Health Symptoms	Current mental condition symptom severity
Complications and Life Threat	Risk of physical complications and life threat if case management is stopped	Mental Health Threat	Risk of persistent personal barriers or poor mental condition care if case management is stopped
Social Domain Items		Health System Domain Items	
Job and Leisure	Personal productivity and leisure activities; employed in the last 6 months; function as a caregiver, fulltime parent and/or homemaker; attend school; have leisure activities like hobbies, participation in social groups, regular outings with friends and family	Access to Care	Access to care and services as they relate to insurance coverage, financial responsibility, language, culture, geography; use of the ED instead of establishing a relationship with a physician(s) or another provider(s)

(continued)

TABLE 4.2 Integrated Case Management-Complexity Assessment Grid (*continued*)

Social Domain Items		Health System Domain Items	
Relationships	Healthy relationships; relationship difficulties; ability to maintain relationships with spouse, family, neighbors, friends, coworkers; presence of dysfunctional relationships; physical altercations with others	Treatment Experience	Experiences with doctors, hospitals, or health system
Residential Stability	Residential stability or suitability; ability to meet financial obligations (rent, mortgage, utilities); access to food, clothing, etc.; housing is safe	Getting Needed Services	Logistical ability to get needed care: getting appointments, transportation to/from appointments; use of the ED instead of seeing outpatient providers; seeing providers that accept cultural practices and/or speak the patient's primary language
Social Support	Availability of social support: have help available when needed or wanted from family, friends, coworkers, other social contacts (e.g., church members) or community supports (e.g., peer support, community health worker)	Provider Collaboration	Communication among providers to ensure coordinated care
Social Vulnerability	Risk of work, loss of income, home, and relational support needs if case management is stopped	Health System Deterrents	Risk of continued poor access to and/or coordination of services if case management is stopped

ADL, activities of daily living; ED, emergency department; IADL, instrumental activities of daily living; SMI, serious mental illness.

health: Physical, Psychological, Social, and Health system. Within each domain we examine where a member's risks or strengths may lie. The risk elements have been updated but continue to look at history, status, and future risk or vulnerability. The risk elements (formerly known as "Anchor Points") are scored 0 to 3 with 0 being no risk and 3 being immediate risk. The elements are totaled providing a risk score. The highest possible risk score is 60.

Let us examine the four domains and the updated individual risk elements.

ICM-CAG Domains

Each of the four domains has five risk elements. The elements review history, current status, and future risk relevant to the specific domain. The detail about each risk element and strategies to decrease risk are outlined. For consistency in the scoring of the risk elements, we review the criteria used:

1. Time frames
   a. History
   b. Current status
   c. Future risk

History encompasses the last 5 years. We want to understand challenges the patient has experienced in the more recent past. Knowing he or she had an appendectomy at age 12 is not relevant to his or her health today; but if the patient has been treated for diabetes and heart disease for at least the last 5 years, these are conditions for which additional assessment and management will affect our work with the patient as well as care planning. In the case of mental health history, we examine the patient's entire life: any mental health or behavioral diagnoses, or challenges at any age, impact future risk and vulnerability. For example, a 47-year-old patient may not report any symptoms of depression recently, but at the age of 14 years was very depressed due to bullying at school and was hospitalized for self-mutilation (cutting). This history may impact future risk of recurrence of a depressive condition or disorder. To recap, the historical elements in all four domains look back at the last 5 years, *except for mental health history*, which assesses the patient's lifetime.

Current Status

For the current status and in all domains, we look at the last 30 days: what the patient has experienced in this short time frame. This includes physical and behavioral symptoms, social and care-related challenges.

Vulnerability

Based on what we have learned from history and current status, we look at what level of risk the member may experience over the next 3 to 6 months if case management intervention is discontinued.

Health Domains

Biological Domain

The elements in this domain assess a patient's physical condition(s); duration and severity. How difficult was it to come to a diagnosis? Were significant resources utilized? How severe are the patient's symptoms? Do they result in disability for the patient? Does the patient have the ability to follow a treatment plan? Is there interference from depression, anxiety, health literacy, and the like? Once these are examined and scored, we can determine the level of risk that the patient will likely face in the next 3 to 6 months if case management services and interventions were no longer available to the patient. Our goals related to the biological domain should encompass helping the member understand his or her conditions, how other health domains interfere and affect physical health; what are the barriers preventing improvement? Examining these risk factors will help with implementation of interventions that will help support the patient to learn how to self-manage as much as possible and to each one's individual ability, so that each experiences health stability, improved function, and quality of life.

Let us look at each risk element in the Biological Domain, to gain a better understanding of the information needed to accurately score the risk present and suggested actions.

Chronic Illness

0 = Less than 3 months of physical dysfunction and/or an acute condition
- No action required

1 = More than 3 months of physical dysfunction, or intermittent dysfunction for the past 3 months, that is, pain, loss of appetite
- Review with the patient his or her understanding of why this dysfunction has occurred; the cause of the dysfunction
- Observe over time if the dysfunction becomes a chronic condition
- Ensure that the patient is following up with the primary care or specialty provider

2 = Presence of a chronic disease/illness
- Review with the patient his or her understanding of the condition and treatment

- Assist the patient in simplifying management if it appears needed

- Ensure the patient is keeping medical appointments

- Evaluate control of the condition by reviewing any symptoms and what metrics are regularly completed: for example, for patients with diabetes, when was the last HgA1c completed and the results? for a patient with hypertension, how often is blood pressure checked and what was the most recent reading?

3 = More than one chronic disease/illness

- Complete activities for Risk Level 2

- Customize any actions related to the results of the assessment: for example, the patient has not had an HgA1c in over a year—important to schedule as soon as possible; a member with heart disease who states he has intermittent chest pain—schedule an appointment with the provider as soon as possible, or refer to the emergency department (ED) if having acute symptoms

- Evaluate the number of providers involved in the patient's care and report findings to the treating providers ensuring all are aware

Diagnostic Difficulty

0 = No difficulty with the diagnosis of a condition; diagnosis was made easily, for example, blood pressure has been elevated for 3 months

- No action needed

1 = A diagnosis was arrived at relatively quickly: for example, patient exhibiting flu-like symptoms and a localized rash—blood test revealed ehrlichiosis from a tick bite

- Observe for any changes in the patient's clinical status

2 = Diagnosis made but only after considerable diagnostic workup: for example, patient diagnosed with multiple sclerosis (MS) but only after blood work, MRI, and spinal tap

- Review with the patient his or her understanding of the condition(s), prescribed treatment, what improvements are expected, and over what time frame

- Assess how the patient managed the diagnostic period

- Discuss what we can do to support the patient to experience a positive outcome
- If the patient is having difficulty with the diagnosis, ask if he or she has discussed this with the physician(s) and would the patient like for us as the case manager to communicate his or her concerns

3 = After significant diagnostic workup, no firm diagnosis has been made

- Complete all actions under Risk Level 2 immediately
- Customize any interventions based on what we learn
- Ask the patient what concerns him or her the most about not reaching a diagnosis
- Offer to communicate these concerns to all involved providers

Symptom Severity and Impairment

0 = No physical symptoms or symptoms are resolved by treatment: for example, migraine headaches are controlled by regularly scheduled Botox injections

- No action required other than to observe efficacy of current treatment

1 = Mild symptoms, but do not interfere with daily function: for example, arthritic pain in hands but still able to knit and crochet, able to work in the garden

- Observe for worsening symptoms

2 = Moderate symptoms that interfere with daily functions: for example, chronic back pain that requires rest and analgesics; may miss 1 to 3 days of work

- Ensure primary care and other involved providers are aware of symptoms
- Ensure patient is following up with providers as required
- Be aware of any follow-up testing that may be ordered for worsening symptoms
- Make sure patient understands condition, what to report to providers, when to seek immediate care
- If assistive interventions are required, assist in facilitation and coordination

3 = Severe symptoms that result in an inability to perform many daily functions: for example, patient with chronic obstructive pulmonary

disease (COPD) is unable to climb the stairs to the second floor of his or her home, vacuum the floors, or walk one block to the market; a patient with MS is chair bound and requires assistance to bathe and use the toilet

- Complete actions from Risk Levels 1 and 2 immediately
- Update the patient's providers with any concerns or risks
- Customize other actions based on what was learned from the assessment
- Assess what current interventions help the patient most; what is working
- Assess what is notworking; where challenges lie
- Evaluate the presence of social support that can aid with those activities too difficult for the patient to perform or complete
- Facilitate and coordinate with collaboration from the treating physician, and provide services that might result in comfort or improvement, for example, rehabilitation, home care

Adherence Ability

0 = Ability to follow a treatment plan; the treatment plan is uncomplicated

1 = The treatment plan is slightly complicated but the client can follow it

2 = The treatment plan is slightly complicated but the client has difficulty following; the client needs support and motivation to adhere to it

3 = The client is unable to follow the prescribed treatment plan due to physical symptoms or has behavioral conditions that interfere with the ability to adhere to it

Vulnerability and Life Threat

0 = Little to no risk of worsening physical symptoms and/or limitations in activities of daily living

- No action required

1 = Mild risk of worsening physical symptoms and/or limitations in activities of daily living

- Encourage adherence to treatment and observe for any barriers that may appear
- Work with patient to remove barriers

2 = Moderate risk of worsening physical symptoms and/or substantial limitations in activities of daily living

- Work with the patient to address any causes for nonadherence
- If behavioral conditions are a cause, work to coordinate needed behavioral services
- Ensure patient and provider are communicating and each understands each other's goals and concerns
- Monitor appropriate clinical tests and utilization, for example, blood sugar, blood pressure, blood chemistries, scans, admissions, ED visits, and so forth
- Case management intervention may be intermittent or long term

3 = Severe risk of physical complications associated with permanent loss of function and/or risk of death

- Perform actions under Risk Level 2
- Customize actions based on assessment
- Perform frequent reassessment of physical symptoms and response to prescribed treatment
- Case management intervention will need to continue until risks are reduced or mitigated
- If appropriate, coordinate long-term, palliative, or hospice care

Psychological Domain

In this domain, we examine an individual's ability to adapt and cope with his or her environment, follow a physician's treatment plan, and respond to treatment for psychiatric illnesses that lead to dysfunction and suffering. This also includes substance use disorders and behavioral conditions without the presence of mental illness.

Barriers to Coping

0 = The ability to manage stress, life situations, and health concerns by seeking support or participating in activities that result in relaxation

and satisfaction, for example, seeking medical advice, hobbies, social activities

- No action required

1 = Limited coping skills such as a need for control, denial of illness, irritability

- Help the patient identify stressors and supports for stressful situations
- Encourage counseling to gain insight into positive coping strategies

2 = Impaired coping skills such as chronic complaining, substance use (self-medication) but without serious impact on medical conditions, mental health, or social situation

- Encourage counseling to gain insight into positive coping strategies that may include specific stress-reduction techniques or conflict-resolution training
- Recommend Employee Assistance Program (EAP) for any work-related stressors
- If living arrangements, work location, or social activities seem to be stressful, discuss with patient strategies to change to reduce stressors
- Screen for alcohol abuse if needed
- Consider reaching out to the patient's primary care physician (PCP) if substance/alcohol abuse are of concern or if the patient may benefit from a mental health professional referral

3 = Poor or absent coping skills manifested by destructive behavior like substance abuse/dependence, psychiatric illness, self-mutilation, suicide attempts, failed/failing social relationships

- Perform actions under risk level 2
- Customize actions based on what was learned in the assessment
- Assist in the development of a crisis intervention plan that may include the patient's support system and providers
- Collaborate with providers for a mental health referral for assessment and treatment recommendations

- Support and encourage mental health treatment with the patient
- Collaborate with the PCP for a referral to substance/alcohol abuse treatment
- Support and encourage participation in substance/alcohol abuse treatment

Mental Health History

0 = No history of mental health problems or conditions
- No action required

1 = Mental health problems or conditions, but resolved or without clear effects on daily function
- Encourage regular primary care screenings for mental conditions with intervention, if appropriate
- Check for access to support from mental health professionals

2 = Mental health conditions that have clear effects on daily function, the need for therapy, medication, day treatment, or a partial inpatient program
- Ensure the patient's understanding of potential for recurrence of mental health conditions by using lay language
- Understand the potential for medical and physical condition interactions, if indicated
- Facilitate and coordinate visits and regular follow-up with a psychiatrist and/or mental health team (psychologists, social workers, nurses, substance use disorder and other counselors); provide support when conditions destabilize
- Facilitate, coordinate, and support follow-up with the PCP
- Refer to a medical home, if available, to ensure all needed services are provided in one setting
- Monitor patient symptoms over time (e.g., PHQ-9, GAD-7)
- Assist with communication among physical and mental health–treating clinicians

3 = Psychiatric admissions and/or persistent effects on daily function due to mental illness

- Perform actions under Risk Level 2
- Include customized actions based on interview
- Facilitate communication between the mental health team for mental conditions and with the PCPs who care for concurrent physical illness
- Collaborate with providers to develop transition plans that will prevent readmissions.
- Support, encourage, and assist the patient to make and keep appointments with providers, especially mental health providers
- Facilitate and coordinate any outpatient services ordered by the treating physician to help stabilize the patient's mental illness(es)
- Facilitate and coordinate appropriate social support for the patient to prevent symptom exacerbation and readmission

Resistance to Treatment

0 = Interested in receiving treatment and willing to cooperate actively

- No action required

1 = Some ambivalence or hesitation, though willing to cooperate with prescribed treatment

- Educate patient/family about illnesses
- Initiate discussions with patient about willingness to recognize conditions and prescribed treatments using motivational-interviewing and problem-solving techniques to facilitate change
- Explore other barriers to treatment adherence
- Inform providers of adherence problems and work with them to consider alternative interventions, if needed

2 = Considerable resistance and nonadherence; hostility or indifference toward health care professionals, diagnosed conditions, and/or treatments

- Perform actions under Risk Level 1

- Actively explore and attempt to reverse other sources of resistance (e.g., family member's negativism, religious objections, cultural influences, relationships with treating physician)

3 = Active resistance to important medical care

- Perform actions under risk levels 1 and 2

- Include customized actions based on interview

- Collaborate with treating clinicians in considering and instituting alternative interventions

- If needed, work with case management medical director to find second opinion practitioners

- If significant resistance exists and is pervasive, consider discontinuation of case management

Mental Health Symptoms

0 = No mental health symptoms

- No action needed

1 = Mild mental health symptoms, such as problems with concentration or feeling tense or nervous but do not interfere with current functioning

- Ensure the patient is receiving primary care treatment with access to support from mental health professionals

- Facilitate communication between all treating providers

2 = Moderate mental health symptoms, such as anxiety, depression, or mild cognitive impairment that interfere with current functioning

- Perform actions under risk level 1

- Ensure that acute maintenance and continuation of treatment is being provided by PCPs with mental health support

- Facilitate primary maintenance and continuation of treatment provided by PCP in a medical home if possible, with mental health specialist assistance—that is, a psychiatrist and mental health team (psychologists, social workers, nurses, substance abuse counselors, et al.)—when condition destabilizes, becomes complicated, or demonstrates treatment resistance

- Evaluate and assess symptoms and document using the PHQ-9, GAD-7, and patient report; report concerns to providers
- Develop a crisis plan with the patient and with provider input

3 = Severe psychiatric symptoms and/or behavioral disturbances, such as violence, self-inflicted harm, delirium, criminal behavior, psychosis, or mania

- Perform actions under risk levels 1 and 2
- Include customized actions based on interview
- Support active and aggressive treatment for mental conditions by a mental health team working in close collaboration with PCPs, who care for concurrent physical illnesses
- When possible, encourage geographically collocated physicaland mental health personnel to facilitate ease of coordinating treatment; for example, medical home or practices in the same vicinity
- Evaluate and assess symptoms and document using the PHQ-9, GAD-7, and patient report; report any concerns immediately to providers

Mental Health Risk and Vulnerability

0 = No evidence of risk

1 = Mild risk of worsening mental health/behavioral symptoms

- Facilitate and coordinate access to appropriate mental health supports and services
- Support and encourage follow-up care with providers and perform intermittent mental health assessments, to monitor symptoms, for example, PHQ-9, GAD-7
- Encourage and support coping and stress reduction activates; can be formal or informal

2 = Moderate risk of worsening mental health symptoms

- Perform actions under risk level 1
- Assist the patient in knowing where and from whom to get assistance: PCP, psychiatrist, counselor, and the like
- Assess symptoms related to depression and anxiety by using tools such as PHQ-9, GAD-7

- Facilitate communication between medical and behavioral providers as necessary; facilitate access to an integrated medical home if possible
- Promote and encourage adherence to prescribed treatment
- Involve caregivers of the patient if agreeable and receive consent in all activities

3 = Severe and persistent risk of psychiatric disorder with frequent health service use

- Perform actions under risk levels 1 and 2
- Include interventions that are specific to the patient's prescribed treatment: medication, therapy, or other more aggressive interventions
- Work with the patient's clinicians to understand the clinical goals and assist the patient with understanding and with removal of barriers to achieve goals
- Patient may need long-term case management involvement

Social Domain

In the social domain, we assess the patient's safety, support, and independence. We look at the presence of a job or school, the ability to meet financial obligations, a safe living environment, support when needed, and the quality of social relationships. Addressing health needs becomes significantly more of a challenge if social supports are lacking or absent.

Job and Leisure

0 = Patient has a "job" which includes employment, furthering education, stay-at-home parent or homemaker, leisure activates that include clubs, hobbies, travel, sports

- No action required

1 = Patient has a job (as described previously) but without leisure activities

- Discuss with the patient past experiences with leisure activity

2 = Patient has leisure activates but does not have a job now or for the last 6 months

- Discuss with member his/her ability to work, willingness to work, or to go to school
- Make referrals to appropriate resources; Social Security for disability, Social Services for educational and vocational resources
- If unable to return to work, provide information on how to access public assistance programs
- Follow up in a timely way to ensure the patient has been able to access any needed resources and assist as necessary
- Encourage any interest in leisure activities

3 = No job for more than 6 months and without leisure activities

- Perform activities under Risk Levels 1 and 2
- Explore the impact of not having a job and income in ability to access health services
- Access to public assistance may be more of an urgency; look for community resources that could assist in the interim

Relationships

0 = No social disruptions; no dysfunctional relationships

1 = Mild social disruptions or interpersonal problems; arguing with family or friends but usually resolving differences with time

- If possible, observe the patient's interactions with family or providers

2= Moderate social dysfunction, social relationships are tenuous, no strong friendships or family ties, would rather be alone

- Encourage member to include family or other supporting acquaintances to be involved in care
- Assess if social issues have any impact on the patient's health, for example, has no one to call when sick
- Assess if the patient is open to work with a counselor to improve social skills
- Explore with the patient if there are social activities in which he or she might be willing to participate

3 = Severe social dysfunction, social isolation, unable to "get along" with family, friends, coworkers, neighbors; argumentative, hostile

- Complete actions from Risk Levels 1 and 2
- Facilitate behavioral health assessment due to disruptive and/or destructive behaviors

Residential Stability

0 = Stable housing, stable living arrangements, able to live independently

- No action required

1 = Stable housing with support of others, for example, family available to assist, receiving home care or home- and community-based services, or living in an institutional setting like assisted living, group home, or long-term care facility

- Facilitate and coordinate additional support where and when needed; this may require looking for community supports, when services are not reimbursed, for example, church volunteers, extended family, friends or coworkers willing to provide support
- Make frequent assessments for potential changes in the patient's needs

2 = Unstable housing, for example, no support at home or living in a shelter; inability to meet financial obligations related to housing; a need to change the current housing situation

- Consult with social services or community housing resources to explore housing options
- Consult with social services or community resources to assist with meeting financial obligations; explore with member the willingness to include family and friends in providing more support
- Be timely with follow-up on availability and coordination of needed resources

3 = No current satisfactory or safe housing, for example, homeless, transient housing (coach surfing), or dangerous environment; an immediate change required

- Immediately connect the patient with safe housing, for example, emergency shelter or shelter with trusted individual
- Follow up with options as soon as the patient is safe for safe housing: consult with social services and/or community housing resources
- Follow-up on coordination of safe housing is a prioritized action
- If appropriate, contact housing authority for needed repairs or mitigation of other unsafe living situations unrelated to violence, for example, vermin or insect infestations, unsafe structures

Social Support

0 = Assistance is readily available from family, friends, coworkers, acquaintances (e.g., church or club members), always
- No action required

1 = Assistance is generally available from family, friends, coworkers, or acquaintances but may be sporadic and not always available when needed
- Assess what assistance is needed
- Discuss with patient and social supports, who can assist and when
- Develop contingency plan for assistance when no one is available: for example, transportation to appointments, what to do in an emergency

2 = Limited assistance from family, friends, coworkers, acquaintances; for example, family does not live close, patient has a limited social circle
- Discuss with patient and social supports, who can assist and when
- Develop contingency plan for assistance when no one is available: for example, transportation to appointments, what to do in an emergency
- Assess for in-home support by home health agencies or volunteer organizations if appropriate

3 = No assistance available from family, friends, coworkers, acquaintances at any time
- Assess for the need and availability of in-home supports, for example, home and community-based services
- Coordinate needed transportation, access to food

- Discuss with patient and providers the need for transfer to a setting that will provide more safety and support, for example, assisted living, group home.

Social Vulnerability

0 = No risk present that warrants the need to change the living situation, social supports are present, and the patient can meet financial obligations.

- No action required

1 = Some assistance might be needed to ensure social supports are available when needed

- Work with member to determine if current supports will be available in the future

- If in-home supports are needed, determine the length of time needed and availability of the services for that period

- Make sure contingency plan is developed for long-term use

2 = Risk exists that would result in the patient having little to no social support, will be unable to meet financial obligations, or keep medical appointments

- Work with the patient and support system to determine if support will continue regardless of how limited support may be

- Explore availability of community and social resources to assist with financial obligations, access to food, and so forth: Is there a limit to what can be accessed?

- Review benefits/reimbursement to ensure any coordinated services can be extended long term

- If unable to extend in-home services, community resources and social support, explore placement options

3 = Immediate, and into the next few months, there is a need for placement of supports, assistance with meeting financial obligations, emergency planning, and/or placement in a safe environment.

- All actions under Risk Level 2 need to be completed as soon as possible

- Expedite placement to a safe environment if home-based options are not feasible

Health System Domain

We often believe if an individual gets the right diagnosis and prescribed treatment, there is no reason to believe his or her health will not improve. But we have often paid no heed to an individual's challenges in getting needed services. In this domain, we examine where and how a patient accesses care. Do they have resources for reimbursement, and do they have faith and trust in their providers? Trust in the health care providers' ability to navigate the system directly impacts health.

Access to Care

0 = Adequate access to care: no issues with insurance, reasonable premiums, co-insurance, co-pays; providers are available near the patient, the patient can make and keep appointments

- No action required

1 = Some difficulty accessing care; long travel to providers; limited access to specialists like psychiatrists; long waits to get appointments; high pharmacy co-pays; providers who meet preferred cultural practice of language not available

- Assist the patient in researching providers who meet their preferences for culture or language

- Assist patients in making appointments

- Discuss medications with high co-pays with pharmacy staff or medical director to see if peer-to-peer could result in more affordable medication

2 = Difficulty accessing care due to geography, language, culture, insurance coverage, or premiums (See detail in #1.)

- All activities in #1 should be completed but with the case manager taking a more active role in helping the patient locate the preferred providers

- Speak with provider offices to facilitate expedited appointments or coordinate multiple appointments in 1 day so that travel is reduced

- Assist with filling gaps in care, for example, lack of counselors: Facilitate telephone, Skype, or other telecommunications for access to counseling services

- If insurance costs are too high, explore what other options may be available to the patient

3 = No adequate access to care due to geography, language, culture, insurance coverage, or premiums (See details in #1)

- Expedite activities in #2
- Contact social services to see if the patient might qualify for access to specialty clinics

Treatment Experience

0 = No problems with health care providers

- No action required

1 = Negative experiences with health care providers

- Ask the patient to describe the experiences
- Ask the patient if he or she could follow the recommended treatment plans
- Ask the patient to describe what kind of provider he or she would like to see
- Help the patient better prepare for provider visits by helping the patient develop questions to ask the provider; recommend the patient write down the questions to take to appointments

2 = Multiple providers; changed providers many times due to dissatisfaction or sees multiple providers

- Complete the actions in #1
- Have the patient describe the conflicts and then assist the patient in resolving conflicts with practitioners if possible by communicating the patient's concerns to the provider
- Review the recommended treatment plan with the patient; ask if this is a plan he or she can follow; if not, why not; facilitate communication of those concerns to the provider
- If conflicts do seem to be resolved, ask the medical director to speak with the provider
- If the patient is still not happy with the provider, help the patient find a new provider

3 = Repeated provider conflicts; ED use

- Complete actions under #2
- Speak with providers to see if a mental health evaluation is warranted
- Offer to coordinate conflict resolution–training and strategies for the patient

Getting Needed Services

Easily available treating practitioners and health care settings (general medical or mental health care); money for medications and medical equipment

0 = No difficulty getting services
1 = Some difficulties in getting to appointments or needed services
- explore barriers preventing access
- coordinate and facilitate the services need to ensure adequate access

2 = Routine difficulties in coordinating and/or getting to appointments or needed services
- assist patient in getting appointments when convenient
- facilitate consistent transportation
- facilitate referrals to specialists
- facilitate needed mental health service when appropriate

3 = Inability to coordinate and/or get to appointments or needed services
- coordinate all interventions for risk score of 2
- explore available services and resources in the patient's community or nearby

Provider Collaboration

0 = Patient able to communicate effectively with all practitioners and practitioners communicate with each other; there are no problems with coordination of care
- No action required

1 = Primary care practitioner coordinates all care including mental health services; limited communication if patient has more than one practitioner
- Review with patient if mental health practitioner is needed
- Communicate with PCP that mental health professional services can be coordinated
- Make the patient aware that integrated practices are available: for example, patient-centered medical home (PCMH) or health home
- Facilitate communication between practitioners and provide medication lists, appointment dates, and so forth

2 = Lack of communication among providers related to a patient's conditions and ordered treatment

- Implement actions under #1
- Help the patient schedule same-day appointments for different problems. Patient can be instructed to bring summary of each visit to the next session
- Communicate with all practitioners that you can facilitate coordination of needed care and services
- Suggest accessing care at an integrated clinic (e.g., PCMH or health home)

3 = No communication among providers and no responsible party for care coordination

- Implement all actions under #2
- Attend provider visits with the patient if possible
- Speak with treating practitioners on behalf of the patient, with the patient's permission (may need to have written consent)

Health System Deterrents/Vulnerability

0 = No risk or concern that care between medical and behavioral is not coordinated; no issues with insurance or financial

- No action required

1 = Mild risk of health system challenges such as insurance coverage restrictions, geographical access to care, inconsistent or limited communication between providers, or inconsistent coordination of care

- Examine with the patient any insurance coverage restrictions or deterrents like high deductible, or co-insurance, exclusions
- Investigate community resources for services not covered by insurance, for example, counseling, other mental health services
- Determine with the patient if he or she has the resources to maintain insurance coverage
- If there is a threat to maintaining coverage, strategize how to mitigate that threat
- Is it possible for the patient to continue to see providers who are not geographically convenient?
- Continue to facilitate communication between providers

2 = Moderate risk of health system challenges related to insurance coverage restrictions, potential loss of insurance coverage, geographical access to care, poor communication among providers, and poor care coordination

- Complete actions in #1
- Assist with finding resources to continue affordable health insurance coverage if unable to maintain current coverage
- Facilitate care in a medical home to improve communication and care coordination

3 = Severe risk of health system challenges such as no health insurance, limited coverage, providers resistant to communication, and no obvious coordination of care

- Complete actions in Risk Levels 1 and 2 immediately

Now let us apply the ICM-CAG to an assessment:

CASE STUDY

Randy is a 45-year-old construction worker admitted to the hospital 2 weeks ago with chest pain and shortness of breath. Randy is single, lives with his elderly, frail mother, and has been laid off work for 3 months. He was diagnosed with hypertension and atrial fibrillation 4 years ago. He is morbidly obese with a body mass index (BMI) of 42. During this recent admission, Randy required cardioversion uncontrolled atrial fibrillation, was newly diagnosed with type II diabetes, congestive heart failure, and central sleep apnea. Randy's blood sugar on admission was 600; he had significant edema in his lower extremities and elevated brain natriuretic peptide (BNP). Two sleep studies were required to diagnose the central sleep apnea. Cardiac testing during the admission revealed a low ejection fraction. He was able to ambulate only 50 to 75 feet on admission, but is now able to ambulate 100 to 150 feet without getting short of breath. Randy's length of stay (LOS) was 10 days. He was discharged on insulin, with instructions to test his blood sugar at least twice per day, to follow up with his PCP in 7 days, and to see a cardiologist. A BiPap was ordered for Randy to use during sleep. Randy did not receive insulin and testing supplies for 3 days after discharging due to poor communication between the patient and the hospital. Randy did not understand that he had to take the prescriptions to the pharmacy to be filled; he thought the hospital had already sent the orders. Randy called the university clinic but they had no record of his discharge orders.

Randy does not have a history of any mental or behavioral conditions. He does, however, seem to be a bit nonchalant about recent health events. Randy shared that his dad had diabetes and "it was no big deal." It is important to note that Randy's father passed away from renal failure as a result of his diabetes. He also shared that he wants to return to work.

Randy's line of work is very physical, carrying heavy loads, shoveling and transporting rock, working in the elements, and the like. He does not seem to have a good understanding about the seriousness of his conditions.

As stated earlier, Randy has been laid off work for the last 3 months. He has been a member of a bowling team for the last 10 years with the same teammates. He has a sister in town but she is a single mother working two part-time jobs. Randy lives with his mother, who owns

Date:	HEALTH RISKS AND HEALTH NEEDS						
Name: Randy	HISTORICAL		CURRENT STATE		VULNERABILITY	
Total Score = 38	Complexity Item	Score	Complexity Item	Score	Complexity Item	Score
Biological Domain	Chronic Illness	3	Symptom Severity/ Impairment	3	Complications and Life Threat	3
	Diagnostic Difficulty	2	Adherence Ability	3		
Psychological Domain	Barriers to Coping	1	Resistance to Treatment	2	Mental Health Threat	2
	Mental Health History	0	Mental Health Symptoms	0		
Social Domain	Job and Leisure	1	Residential Stability	1	Social Vulnerability	3
	Relationships	0	Social Support	2		
Health System Domain	Access to Care	1	Getting Needed Services	3	Health System Deterrents	3
	Treatment Experience	2	Provider Collaboration	3		

Scoring System
Green   0 = no vulnerability or need to act
Yellow   1 = mild vulnerability and need for monitoring or prevention
Orange   2 = moderate vulnerability and need for action or development of intervention plan
Red   3 = severe vulnerability and need for immediate action or immediate intervention plan

the home, and he is a caregiver for his mother, helping with cooking, household chores, and transportation.

Randy has always accessed care at the university clinic where his mother seeks care; the clinic is 50 miles from his residence. Randy never sees the same physician twice as the clinic is staffed by medical school residents. Randy's mother is a Medicare and Medicaid recipient and has always sought care at the clinic. Even though Randy has health coverage through his union, he has continued to attend the clinic because he was responsible for getting his mother to her appointments. Randy's current health coverage will expire in 2 months due to the time off work. He has the option of paying Consolidated Omnibus Budget Reconciliation Act (COBRA) insurance for a time, but will need to eventually find another method of health coverage.

Rationale for Scoring

Please review the reasons for which the documented risk scores were applied to the ICM-CAG based on the information learned from Randy's assessment.

Biological Domain

Chronic Illness Score = 3: Randy has a 4-year history of hypertension and atrial fibrillation.

Two weeks ago, he was diagnosed with diabetes, heart failure, and central sleep apnea during the recent admission; a high BMI resulted in a diagnosis of morbid obesity.

Diagnostic Difficulty Score = 2: Two sleep studies were conducted to diagnose the central sleep apnea. This condition differs from obstructive sleep apnea but causes the same complications. The diabetes was not diagnosed before this admission which makes us concerned that this may have been missed during any previous clinic visits.

Symptom Severity Score = 3: Randy had shortness of breath and chest pain which resulted in the recent admission. He also is limited in ambulation because of these symptoms which are considered severe.

Adherence Ability Score = 3: Randy appears to have a poor understanding of the seriousness of his condition that contributes to his inability to adhere to a treatment plan. The seriousness of his conditions will require behavioral changes to improve: changing diet, increasing activity, follow-up visits, and medication.

Complications and Life Threat Score = 3: Without the assistance of case management, Randy's chronic conditions will likely continue to be uncontrolled. The severity of his current conditions could lead to severe disability or death.

Psychological Domain

Barriers to Coping Score = 1: While Randy does not necessarily have obvious coping deficits, his history of chronic conditions and resulting increase in symptoms leading to the recent admission tell us he has a lack of insight and understanding of the seriousness of his conditions.

Mental Health History Score = 0: Randy has no history of mental illness.

Resistance to Treatment Score = 3: Worsening health indicates Randy has not taken steps to control his conditions. The resistance to treatment may not be conscious or intentional, but regardless, not following prescribed treatment has led to his current compromised health.

Mental Health Symptoms Score = 0: Randy exhibits no symptoms of any mental or behavioral conditions.

Mental Health Threat Score = 2: This score may be surprising, but if we think about the potential for worsening health over the next 3 to 6 months, without case management support and interventions, Randy will not understand how serious his health conditions are which would result in worsening health and increased worry and concern which will result in the inability to cope with worsening health. His lack of understanding, or laissez-faire approach to health, will prevent improvement.

Social Domain

Job and Leisure Score = 1: Randy has been off work for 3 months and has participated in leisure activities being a longtime member of a bowling team. Randy has a personal goal of returning to work.

Relationships Score = 0: There is no evidence that Randy has any difficulties with developing or maintaining relationships.

Residential Stability Score = 1: Randy lives with his mother who owns the home. However, because he is out of work, there is a potential that it may be difficult to pay for living expenses.

Social Support Score = 2: Randy is his frail, elderly mother's primary caregiver and his sister has limited ability to assist. Randy has his bowling team friends but we do not yet know if any of them are available to assist Randy if needed. There is no plan in place should Randy's health decline.

Social Vulnerability Score = 3: There are serious concerns about what will happen because Randy will likely be unable to return to work any time soon, if ever. Will he have needed financial resources to buy food, pay utilities, and so forth? Since he is the primary caregiver for his mother, if his health worsens, who will care for her and be there to assist him?

Health System Domain

Access to Care Score = 1: Randy has had good health coverage and access to providers nearby but has chosen to seek care from a university clinic 50 miles away. However, his coverage will end in a couple of months.

Treatment Experience Score = 1: Randy has seen a different practitioner with nearly every visit to the clinic. This has likely contributed to the poor management of his conditions.

Getting Needed Services Score = 3: Randy has access to care but has chosen to seek care at the university clinic where his mother seeks care. His recent decline in health, specifically the diagnosis of significantly uncontrolled diabetes, is likely due to inconsistent care and communication by the clinic staff.

Provider Collaboration Score = 3: It is unclear if the discharge orders were received by the university clinic. Randy did not receive needed supplies or instructions and even when he called the clinic, it seemed they were unaware of his discharge needs.

Health System Deterrents Score = 3: Randy is at significant risk of worsening health unless the case manager can assist him in maintaining insurance coverage. His health will likely not improve without assistance from providers who better communicate and address his needs. He will need to access a PCP and appropriate specialists closer to his home. ■ ■ ■

REFERENCE

Kathol, R. G., Perez, R., & Cohen, J. S. (2010). *The integrated case management manual: Assisting complex patients regain physical and mental health.* New York, NY: Springer Publishing.

CHAPTER 5

Assessing the Pediatric Patient Using the Integrated Case Management Complexity Assessment Grid

Rebecca Perez
Kathleen Fraser

Love every child without condition, listen with an open heart, get to know who they are, what they love, and follow more often than you lead.

—Adele Devine, *Flying Starts for Unique Children: Top Tips for Supporting Children With SEN or Autism When They Start School*

OBJECTIVES

- Understand the Integrated Case Management (ICM) process for children/adolescents with health complexities
- Understand the similarities and differences between the adult and pediatric complexity assessment grids
- Understand the need for assessment of family issues related to pediatric caregiving
- Understand the professional case manager's actions with the scores and a patient-centered plan of care
- Understand nursing documentation related to the ICM process

Adults are not exclusive in experiencing complexity. Pediatric patients can experience complexity as well, but our approach to support them is very different from that of the adult. As a result, the Case Management Society of America (CMSA) developed a version of the Integrated Complexity Assessment Grid for use with children and youth. This chapter outlines how best to address the risks that exist for children and adolescents experiencing complex medical and behavioral conditions that may be further complicated by social and health system barriers. Pediatric-integrated case management (PICM) follows the same standards of practice for case management. However, there exist unique challenges when assisting children/youth and their families with health complexity in addition to also having to consider the contributions of caregivers/parents, teachers, coaches, and peers in their child-specific assessments and care plan development. Children/youth are at as great a risk for multiple factors contributing to health complexity as adults; therefore, an approach to integrated pediatric case management parallels the approach taken with adults. This will allow case management programs that understand the importance of correcting mental health issues as a means of reversing persistent physical symptoms to include a child/youth component in their case management services, particularly if they have already decided to provide adult-integrated case management and have a child/youth population to serve as well.

Basics of the Pediatric-Integrated Case Management Complexity Assessment Grid

The pediatric version of the Integrated Case Management Complexity Assessment Grid (PIM-CAG) was originally developed with input from pediatric psychiatrists, pediatricians, child psychologists, and pediatric case managers under the guidance of the developers of the original Integrated Case Management Complexity Assessment Grid (IM-CAG). You will notice some overlap between the Adult CAG and the Pediatric CAG, but additional risk elements have been added to the PIM-CAG to be inclusive of the special needs of the child and adolescent. Like the ICM-CAG, the PIM-CAG is specifically developed for use by case managers rather than by treating practitioners. Once again, we emphasize that the role of case managers is to uncover barriers to improvement, coordinate care and services, advocate and support the patient so that he or she can eventually reach a level of self-management. It is not our role to diagnose or treat, so it is not necessary to know all physical or mental health interventions that may be involved. With assessment and use of the PIM-CAG, we can identify the barriers preventing health improvement and work with the patient (if appropriate), family, guardian, or caregiver in obtaining the necessary care and services that will impact the child's health and well-being. As with adults, one item could trigger multiple actions by the case manager involving more than one health domain. The PIM-CAG is used not only as a prioritization of needed interventions, it can also be used as a communication tool to be shared with the child's support system as well as providers.

The PIM-CAG goes far beyond assessing risks in physical and mental health. It includes factors that influence the ability of the child or adolescent to maximize his or her health by assessing cognitive functioning, family relationships, relationships with friends, school experience, adverse life events, and the health and abilities of the parent/caregiver. What is most important to understand is that our approach to working with children and adolescents must be different. Children and adolescents are not small adults; their world view is very different; their needs are very different. So must be our approach to be helpful and effective.

Similarities and Differences Between the PIM-CAG and the IM-CAG

Like the ICM-CAG, the PIM-CAG is used to conduct an integrated case management assessment since it provides a method through which illness and life situation complexity can be prioritized by assigning levels of risk and then acted upon on behalf of the child/adolescent. We will review the risk elements as they pertain to the child and adolescent. For those who may be providing case management intervention to this population but are less familiar with conditions and challenges of the pediatric population, we encourage you to review Chapter 3 to learn more about behavioral challenges in children and then make sure you are familiar with how medical conditions are treated. Diabetes in a child will have nuances not found in the treatment of adults. Pediatric cancers and hematological disorders also are treated differently than in adults. For an adult, chemotherapy may be administered in the outpatient setting, but a child may require an acute care admission to receive treatment. Remember it is your professional responsibility to understand the conditions your patients face.

An additional caveat to working with the pediatric population is the need to focus on parents, guardians, and caregivers. If the individuals responsible for the health and well-being of the child are not functionally capable of meeting the child's needs, you may have some very difficult interventions to consider. The parent/guardian/caregiver may need the interventions of a case manager for assistance in managing their own challenges so that they can be a support to the child. You may also find parents/guardians/caregivers who are not providing a safe environment for the child; perhaps the child is in danger of injury; you will be required to report to authorities these concerns. This can be uncomfortable, especially if you have been working with the child's support system for some time. Ultimately, the child is your patient, and you must always act in the child's best interest.

The Child/Adolescent and Caregivers/Parents Interview and Assessment

Integrated case management is based on the relationship developed between the case manager and the patient to support health improvement and reduce impairment. The PIM-CAG is scored similar to the ICM-CAG based on the assessment discussion with the parent/guardian/caregiver. Depending on the child, age, and parental consent, the child may participate in the assessment and care-planning processes. For adolescents, they should be part of the assessment discussion in so far as they can understand the issues and parents are accepting of the inclusion.

As part of the usual process, the case manager should review any clinical notes and/or claims information available about the child/youth. One most important task to complete before working with any child or adolescent is to determine who the legal guardians are, then define any issues related to confidentiality and how they will be honored, and determine the expectations of the parent/guardian and child or adolescent. Are there any issues with parental relationships like separation or divorce, custody, or disagreements about how to address the child's needs? If the patient is an adolescent, how will you work with the parent/guardian when the adolescent wishes to participate in his or her care? Parents/guardians may want to shield the child/adolescent from worry. Negotiation with all concerned needs to occur to ensure participation and engagement in case management

TABLE 5.1 Pediatric Integrated Case Management Assessment Grid Scoring Sheet

Date:	HEALTH RISKS AND HEALTH NEEDS					
Name:	HISTORICAL		CURRENT STATE		VULNERABILITY	
Total Score =	Complexity Item	Score	Complexity Item	Score	Complexity Item	Score
Biological Domain	Chronic Illness		Symptom Severity/ Impairment		Complications and Life Threat	
	Diagnostic Difficulty		Adherence Ability			
Psychological Domain	Barriers to Coping		Resistance to Treatment		Learning and/ or Mental Health Threat	
	Mental Health History		Mental Health Symptoms			
	Cognitive Development					
	Adverse Developmental Events					
Social Domain	Learning Ability		Residential Stability		Family/School/ Social System Vulnerability	
	Family and Social Relationships		Child/Adolescent Support System			
	Caregiver/ Parent Health and Function		Caregiver/Family Support			
			School and Community Participation			
Health System Domain	Access to Care		Getting Needed Services		Health System Deterrents	
	Treatment Experience		Provider Collaboration			

Scoring System
Green: 0 = no vulnerability or need to act
Yellow: 1 = mild vulnerability and need for monitoring or prevention
Orange: 2 = moderate vulnerability and need for action or development of intervention plan
Red: 3 = severe vulnerability and need for immediate action or immediate intervention plan

(continued)

TABLE 5.1 Pediatric Integrated Case Management Assessment Grid Scoring Sheet (*continued*)

Date:	HEALTH RISKS AND HEALTH NEEDS		
Name:	HISTORICAL	CURRENT STATE	VULNERABILITY
Biological Domain Items		Psychological Domain Items	
Chronic Illness	Presence of chronic physical illness	Barriers to Coping	Problems handling stress or engaging in problem solving
		Mental Health History	Prior mental condition
Diagnostic Difficulty	Difficulty getting a condition diagnosed; multiple providers have been consulted; multiple diagnostic tests completed	Cognitive Development	Cognitive level and capabilities
		Adverse Developmental Events	Early adverse physical and mental health events: complications during pregnancy; other adverse event that took place early in childhood resulting in interrupting cognitive or behavioral development; trauma
Symptom Severity/ Impairment	Physical illness symptom severity and impairment; do the physical symptoms result in a disability, i.e., unable to care for self, ADL, IADL; unable to attend school or participate in any school-related activity, e.g., physical education	Resistance to Treatment	Resistance to treatment; nonadherence; encompasses the parent/guardian and/or the child/adolescent: doesn't believe the treatment is right for him/her; not following a physician's treatment plan due to poor health, poor health literacy, lack of understanding related to the goal of treatment; a behavioral condition has interfered, e.g., depression, anxiety, poorly managed SMI
Adherence Ability	Current difficulties in the ability to follow a physician's treatment plan by the parent/ guardian or the child	Mental Health Symptoms	Current mental conditions with symptom severity; presence of mental health symptoms or challenging behaviors
Complications and Life Threat	Risk of physical complications and life threat if case management is stopped	Learning and/ or Mental Health Threat	Risk of persistent personal barriers, cognitive deficits, or poor mental condition care if case management is stopped

(*continued*)

TABLE 5.1 Pediatric Integrated Case Management Assessment Grid Scoring Sheet (*continued*)

Date:	HEALTH RISKS AND HEALTH NEEDS		
Name:	HISTORICAL	CURRENT STATE	VULNERABILITY
Social Domain Items		Health System Domain Items	
Learning Ability	History/presence of learning difficulties, ability to participate in learning activities	Access to Care	Access to care and services as they relate to insurance coverage, financial responsibility, language, geography; use of the ED instead of establishing a relationship with a physician or other provider
Family and Social Relationships	Stability in parent/ guardian relationships; ability to make friends, socialize with peers		
Caregiver Health and Function	Caregiver/parent physical and mental health condition and function; ability to support the health and well-being of the child/adolescent	Treatment Experience	Experience with doctors, hospitals, or other areas of the health system
Residential Stability	Food and housing situation; safe place to live, free from abuse, neglect; resources are available to support safe living, financial resources for food, utilities, rent, mortgage	Getting Needed Services	Logistical ability to get needed care: getting appointments, use of the ED instead of seeking outpatient care
Child/ Adolescent Support System	Child/youth support system, who is available to support the child?		
Caregiver/ Family Support System	Caregiver/parent support system; who provides social support to family/caregiver?	Provider Collaboration	Communication among providers to ensure coordinated care
School and Community Participation	Attendance, achievement, and behavior at school		
Family/ School/Social Vulnerability	Risk for home/school support or supervision needs if case management is stopped	Health System Deterrents	Risk of continued poor access to and/or coordination of services if case management is stopped

ADL, activities of daily living; ED, emergency department; IADL, instrumental activities of daily living; SMI, serious mental illness.

intervention. Very young children will not likely be involved in the assessment and care-planning process. Older children and adolescents may wish to participate and the negotiation that must take place includes what the parent/guardian is comfortable with the child knowing, and how much autonomy will be afforded to the child/adolescent. It is natural for parents and caregivers to want to protect, but we can also help them understand that taking responsibility for one's health cannot start too soon. Allowing the child/adolescent to be actively involved in his or her health will result in improved self-management as he or she grows and matures. We must be sensitive to an adolescent's developing independence. Some may welcome complete transparency with the parent/guardian while others may want to keep some information confidential. At the beginning of the relationship development, the parent/guardian and patient need to understand that information that may be harmful or helpful will be disclosed only as appropriate. States may have very specific laws and regulations related to the age of consent or how information should be shared between parent/guardian and patient. You must make yourself aware of and familiar with the laws in the jurisdiction in which you practice.

Children and adolescents experiencing health complexity will likely need long-term case management intervention. The assessment process may take even more time than we would typically see with the complex adult patient. It may take more time to understand the relationships between the patient, parent/guardians, other family members, providers, school, and friends. While more effort is required by the case manager, relationship development will likely be more successful and is necessary to be effective in assisting the child/adolescent to move toward improved health.

The PIM-CAG contains 25 items in four domains, whereas the IM-CAG contains 20 items in four domains. The scoring range for the PIM-CAG, therefore, is from 0 to 75 while the scoring range for the IM-CAG is from 0 to 60. You will notice that risk elements in the social domain are expanded to address the special needs of the child/adolescent. Risk scoring remains the same; however, the time frames differ for this population. Historical items will examine the child/adolescent's entire life except for "Access to Care" which examines the last 6 months. Current risk elements will examine the last 30 days.

Future risk/vulnerability will examine the next 3 to 6 months just as the Adult CAG.

The five new items that have been added to the PIM-CAG include: Cognitive Development, Adverse Developmental Events, School Functioning, Caregiver/Parent Health and Function, and Child/Youth Support. These five items recognize and capture the complexity that may be experienced by children and adolescents.

While cognitive deficits can occur in adults (e.g., various dementias), these differ in the child or adolescent. This risk element encompasses the presence of intellectual disabilities, as well as the spectrum of developmental disorders like autism, or pervasive developmental disorder. Children and adolescents with deficits in cognitive development may need specialized educational settings, support personnel in the home, and assistance with socialization since development delay is not understood and is often handled ineffectively due to lack of understanding by nonprofessionals.

Adverse Developmental Events has been added to the Psychological Domain to bring awareness of both physical and behavioral exposures that have historically impacted, or may impact in the future, cognitive abilities, emotions, or behaviors. These include, but are not limited to, toxic exposures like lead, traumatic brain injuries, trauma such as physical or psychological abuse and neglect, or other central nervous system illnesses that may occur because of birth trauma, like cerebral palsy. While some of the adverse events are the result of a physical or biological event, we typically see a greater risk in behavioral or mental illness symptoms. If there are coexisting physical symptoms or conditions, these can be captured in the Biological Domain.

Children and adolescents do not work in the traditional sense—their "work" is attending school and participating in school and community activities like school clubs, sports, Boy and Girl Scouts, 4 H, and so on. The two risk elements added to the assessment are historical School Functioning and current School and Community Participation. We examine school performance that includes their ability to be successful in school, attendance, and behavior at school and with peers. If risk is assessed, we may need to assist in facilitating more involvement by parents/guardians, school administrators, and health providers. Know that past performance in school will be an indicator of future performance.

Caregiver/Parent Health and Function has been added to provide a general assessment of the person(s) responsible for the child or adolescent's health, well-being, and safety. We want to better understand the ability of the parent/guardian to meet the needs of a child or adolescent with complex health needs. If the parent/guardian is incapable of meeting the child's needs, we must facilitate actions and interventions to compensate for any lack of ability on the part of the parent/caregiver. This element demonstrates the strengths of the parent/caregiver, or may indicate the need for more significant intervention to keep a child safe.

Caregiver/Family Support is essentially the same as the ICM-CAG Social Support element. We evaluate who else in the child or adolescent's life can support, mentor, and contribute to the growth and development of the child such as a grandparent or other family member, coach, or teacher who is actively involved in the child's life. We also assess the presence of support in case of emergency or crisis: Who is available to assist the parent/guardian in case of illness or when other urgent/emergent situations arise?

Please refer to the grid in Table 5.1 to guide your risk assessment for the risk elements that mirror the ICM-CAG. Let's examine the risk elements that are unique to the pediatric population and examples of actions to mitigate risk:

Psychological Domain
Cognitive Development

0 = No cognitive impairment
- No action required

1 = Possible developmental delay or immaturity; low IQ
- Assist in establishing level of impairment, including capacity of child to communicate physical needs and symptoms by coordinating referrals for appropriate testing
- Discuss level of impairment and needs with caregivers, educator, and the pediatrician to ensure appropriate placement in school system
- Assess need for remedial educational assistance and home support; facilitate completion of an individual educational plan (IEP) to meet the child's educational needs

- Maintain communication with the school system and medical providers regarding the child's progress with learning

2 = Delayed development; mild or moderate cognitive impairment

- Complete actions under Risk Level 1

- Review performance/adjustment issues with school facility; involve social services if needed if there is a lack of improvement

- Assess and assist with home support for child/youth based on functional capabilities and respite for caregivers/parents related to assimilation of social skills; provide relief for parents/guardians from day-to-day caregiving

- Assess and share child/youth's ability to communicate

3 = Severe and pervasive developmental delays or profound cognitive impairment

- Complete actions under Risk Levels 1 and 2

- Ensure parents/guardian have access to needed resources and supports to deal with severe developmental delays

- In extreme circumstances, placement may be required; ork with providers and parents/guardian to facilitate such a difficult transition

Adverse Developmental Events

0 = No identified developmental traumas or injuries (e.g., physical or sexual abuse, meningitis, lead exposure, drug abuse, exposure to infection, or other untoward prenatal exposures)

- No action required

1 = Traumatic prior experiences or injuries with no apparent or stated impact on child/youth

- While at the time of assessment there may appear to be no untoward effects of early trauma or exposure; observation is warranted as the child grows and develops

2 = Traumatic prior experiences or injuries with potential relationship to impairment in child/youth

- Facilitate needed testing and evaluation for the extent that the trauma or exposure has affected the child

- Facilitate appropriate interventions to reduce the resulting effects of the trauma or exposure

3 = Traumatic prior experiences with apparent and significant direct relationship to impairment in child/youth
- Complete actions under Risk Level 2
- Urgently coordinate needed services to address the impairments experienced due to trauma and exposures

Social Domain
Learning Ability

0 = Performing well in school with good achievement, attendance, and behavior
- No action required

1 = Performing adequately in school although there are some achievement, attendance, and behavioral problems (e.g., missed classes, pranks)
- Encourage parents/caregivers to become more closely involved with the child's teachers and administrators

2 = Experiencing moderate problems with school achievement, attendance, and/or behavior (e.g., school disciplinary action, few school-related peer relationships, academic probation)
- Recommend parents/guardians closely work with teachers and counselors to determine strategies to improve achievement, attendance, and reduce disruptive behavior
- May need to refer to additional counseling or tutoring resources outside of school

3 = Experiencing severe problems with school achievement, attendance, and/or behavior (e.g., homebound education, school suspension, violence, illegal activities at school, academic failure, school dropout, disruptive peer group activity)
- Urgently assist with facilitation of additional resources and referrals for counseling, tutoring

Family and Social Relationships

0 = Stable nurturing home, good social and peer relationships
- No action is required

1 = Mild family problems, minor problems with social and peer relationships (e.g., parent–child conflict, frequent fights, marital discord, lacking close friends)
- Offer to facilitate counseling to address family problems or the child's challenges with making friends

2 = Moderate level of family problems, inability to initiate and maintain social and peer relationships (e.g., parental neglect, difficult separation/divorce, alcohol abuse, hostile caregiver, difficulties in maintaining same-age peer relationships)
- Collaborate with providers and school to encourage family counseling or counseling for the child's inability to maintain relationships
- Involve social services to assess family dysfunction and risk to child/adolescent's safety

3 = Severe family problems with disruptive social and peer relationships (e.g., significant abuse, hostile child custody battles, addiction issues, parental criminality, complete social isolation, little or no association with peers)
- Immediately notify social services or appropriate authorities if there is a risk of danger to the welfare of your patient or other family member
- Notify the patient's providers of concerns with social isolation; facilitate referral to appropriate mental health providers

Caregiver/Parent Health and Function

0 = All caregivers healthy
- No action required

1 = Physical and/or mental health issues, including poor coping skills, and/or permanent disability, present in one or more caregiver, which do not impact parenting

- Discuss with parent/guardian the challenges and contributors to difficulty in coping and what, if any, resources are available to assist with coping
- Assess any needed assistance related to existing disabilities
- Provide resources to the parent/guardian to obtain defined assistance

2 = Physical and/or mental health conditions, including disrupted coping resources, and/or permanent disability, present in one or more caregiver, that interfere with parenting

- Complete actions under Risk Level 1
- Assist parent/guardian in making needed appointments for counseling and other mental health services
- Provide information on resources that may assist the parent/guardian with compensation for any physical disability

3 = Physical and/or mental health conditions, including disrupted coping styles, and/or permanent disability, present in one or more caregiver, which prevent effective parenting and/or create a dangerous situation for the child/youth

- Immediately contact the patient's providers to advise of a dangerous situation
- Work with social services to ensure the patient has a safe environment, even if just temporary
- Reassure the parent/caregiver that you will assist in making sure there is no interruption in the care and services received by the patient

Child/Adolescent Support

0 = Supervision and/or assistance readily available from family/caregiver, friends/peers, teachers, and/or community social networks (e.g., spiritual/religious groups) at all times

- No action required

1 = Supervision and/or assistance generally available from family/caregiver, friends/peers, teachers, and/or community social networks; but possible delays

- Ascertain who besides parent/guardian are able to provide support, caring, and supervision such as friends or teachers
- Create a plan with the parent/caregiver so that these supports are available when needed

2 = Limited supervision and/or assistance available from family/caregiver, friends/peers, teachers, and/or community social networks

- Complete actions under Risk Level 1
- Look for alternative supports, like after-school care or community activities

3 = No effective supervision and/or assistance available from family/caregiver, friends/peers, teachers, and/or community social networks at any time

- Complete actions under Risk Level 2
- Get permission to speak with extended family members to ascertain their ability to support the patient
- Work with school and social services to see what programs might be available to address the patient's need for additional emotional support

School and Community Participation

0 = Attending school regularly, achieving and participating well, and actively engaged in extracurricular school or community activities (e.g., sports, clubs, hobbies, religious groups)

- No action required

1 = Average of 1 day of school missed/week and/or minor disruptions in achievement and behavior with few extracurricular activities

- Discover the reason for missed school days
- Strategize with parent/caregiver on how to prevent missed school days
- Work with parent/guardian and patient to learn what the child is interested in, for example, hobbies, sports, games
- Encourage parent/guardian to connect patient to activities

2 = Average of 2 days or more of school missed/week and/or moderate disruption in achievement or behavior with resistance to extracurricular activities

- Complete actions under Risk Level 1
- Contact patient's school to help facilitate parent/guardian communication with teachers and school counselors to develop plan to improve attendance, performance, and participation

3 = Truant or school nonattendance with no extracurricular activities and no community connections

- Complete actions under Risk Level 1 and 2 with plan for urgent implementation

CASE STUDY

Now let us examine an example of an integrated assessment for a complex pediatric patient (Table 5.2). Danny is an 8-year-old boy currently residing with his second foster family. Danny was placed in the foster care system at age 5 after his mother was sentenced to federal prison on drug-trafficking charges. Danny was diagnosed with attention deficit hyperactivity disorder (ADHD) at age 3 while attending a Head Start Program. At age 6, he was diagnosed with von Willebrand's disease after an injury at school. After this incident, his first foster parent asked that Danny be placed elsewhere because she found his behavior and the new diagnosis of a hematological disorder far too stressful and beyond her capabilities.

Danny has struggled in school due to his ADHD. He is often separated from his class due to disruptive behavior and is extremely active, finding it difficult to sit or be inactive for any length of time. There is also concern that he may have a learning disability as his reading level does not equate to the expected grade level. To date, he has not had any testing. He loves to play outdoors, and play sports, especially football and baseball, but gets very frustrated and angry when he is not allowed to play. He has been to the emergency room three times in the last 6 months due to injuries with one resulting in an admission due to excessive bleeding from a fall at school; the emergeny department (ED) visits addressed large hematomas that occurred while playing football and jumping off a swing. He has required infusion of factors to address hematomas and the bleeding. Danny has a pediatrician and oncologist and his foster family ensures he keeps all appointments. They are interested in getting home infusions for factors rather than going to the hospital or hospital outpatient clinic. He becomes very anxious and agitated when he sees he is going to the hospital. Danny has health coverage through his state's Medicaid program for Children with Special Health Care Needs. There are no concerns with access to needed care and services.

Danny has been with his new foster family for 2 years. Sharon and Bill are committed to Danny and want to provide him with a safe and loving home. They admit his behaviors are challenging and sometimes are overwhelmed because he is so active and they fear that he will continue to injure himself. But their priority is to make sure Danny feels secure and loved and to better address his ADHD so that he can feel successful in school and learn to better control his impulses so that he does not suffer significant injuries. Sharon and Bill would like to see if his needed infusions for factors could be administered at home rather than in the hospital setting and would like to find some additional support outside of school to address his ADHD. At present, Danny is not taking any medication to address ADHD symptoms, but Bill and Sharon wonder if medication might help Danny do better in school. ■ ■ ■

Biological Domain

Chronic Illness = 2: There is presence of a serious medical illness for which there is no cure and which requires immediate intervention

Diagnostic Difficulty = 1: Condition was easily diagnosed after traumatic injury

Symptom Severity = 2: Condition requires urgent intervention when a bleeding event occurs; requires implementation of safety measures to prevent bleeding events

Adherence Ability = 2: Danny's foster parents are able to and do adhere to Danny's treatment plan but Danny's behaviors make it challenging to prevent injury

Complications and Life Threat = 3: Danny requires urgent interventions to prevent life threat. Without case management intervention to assist with needed care coordination, Danny is at risk of death from hemorrhaging

TABLE 5.2 Pediatric Integrated Complexity Assessment Grid Scoring Sheet

Date:	HEALTH RISKS AND HEALTH NEEDS						
Name: Danny	HISTORICAL		CURRENT STATE		VULNERABILITY		
Total Score = 43	Complexity Item	Score	Complexity Item	Score	Complexity Item	Score
Biological Domain	Chronic Illness	2	Symptom Severity/ Impairment	2	Complications and Life Threat	3
	Diagnostic Difficulty	1	Adherence Ability	2		
Psychological Domain	Barriers to Coping	2	Resistance to Treatment	0	Learning and/ or Mental Health Threat	3
	Mental Health History	2				
	Cognitive Development	2	Mental Health Symptoms	2		
	Adverse Developmental Events	2				
Social Domain	Learning Ability	2	Residential Stability	0	Family/School/ Social System Vulnerability	2
	Family and Social Relationships	3	Child/ Adolescent Support System	1		
	Caregiver/ Parent Health and Function	2	Caregiver/ Family Support	1		
			School and Community Participation	2		
Health System Domain	Access to Car	0	Getting Needed Services	2	Health System Deterrents	2
	Treatment Experience	0	Provider Collaboration	0		

Scoring System
Green   0 = no vulnerability or need to act
Yellow   1 = mild vulnerability and need for monitoring or prevention
Orange   2 = moderate vulnerability and need for action or development of intervention plan
Red   3 = severe vulnerability and need for immediate action or immediate intervention plan

Psychological Domain

Barriers to Coping = 2: Danny has exhibited anger and frustration because he is not allowed to play sports. He does not understand why and acts out as a result.

Mental Health History = 2: Danny has been diagnosed with ADHD without any known treatment.

Cognitive Development = 2: Danny's reading level does not equal his school grade level. It appears no testing has been done to assess a learning disability.

Adverse Developmental Events = 2: Danny was removed from his mother's care and custody at age 4 and was placed in the foster care system. It is unknown if Danny's mother used substances during her pregnancy; if so, it could be a contributor to a possible learning disability.

Resistance to Treatment = 0: Danny's foster parents are actively involved in Danny's care and want to be more proactive in addressing his challenges.

Mental Health Symptoms = 2: Danny's lack of attention and hyperactivity have resulted in poor school performance and injury. He is unable to sit quietly for any length of time.

Mental Health Threat = 3: Unless Danny's behaviors are better managed, he is at risk of continued delayed development as well as physical risk.

Social Domain

Learning Ability = 2: Danny's reading level does not equate to the expected school grade level. There is no known learning disability but no testing has occurred.

Family and Social Relationships = 3: The effects of removal from his mother's care at a young age is unknown. He has been in the care of two foster care families in 4 years. His first foster care guardian could not manage his behaviors or medical condition. Any other family connections are unknown.

Caregiver/Parent Health and Function = 2: Danny's mother was convicted of felony drug trafficking and sent to prison; as a result, Danny was placed in the foster care system. His first foster parent could not manage his behavior or medical condition. His current foster parents seem better equipped and prepared to care for him, but this history is essential for any possible future vulnerability.

Residential Stability = 0: Danny's current foster parents are able to meet all his needs for a safe environment.

Caregiver/Family Support =1: Danny's current foster family appears very supportive and caring, but other available supports to Danny are unknown.

School and Community Participation = 2: Danny regularly attends school except for physical health events. He loves to play sports but these are risky activities in his circumstance. Danny has no other known interests or hobbies.

Family/School/Social System Vulnerability = 2: There is need to assist the foster care family to find support for them so that they can continue to care for Danny. In order to improve his school successes, additional resources need to be implemented and there is a need to find social activities that Danny enjoys but do not put him at risk of injury.

Health System Domain

Access to Care = 0: Danny has health coverage through his state's program for children.

Treatment Experience = 0: There is no evidence of negative experiences with providers.

Getting Needed Services = 2: Danny receives the care he needs but his foster parents are interested in reducing ED visits and inpatient (IP) admissions by coordinating infusions of factor at home when needed. Danny has not received any treatment for his ADHD and his foster parents are also interested in exploring treatment options.

Provider Collaboration = 0: There is no evidence that Danny's providers are not in good communication.

Health System Deterrents = 2: Without case management assistance, there may be delays in getting home infusion coordinated and discussions related to ADHD treatment. ■ ■ ■

CHAPTER 6

Common Physical and Mental Health Conditions

Rebecca Perez

Kathleen Fraser

Wellness seeks more than the absence of illness; it searches for new levels of excellence. Beyond any disease-free neutral point, wellness dedicates its efforts to our total well-being—in body, mind, and spirit.

—Greg Anderson

OBJECTIVES

- Understand cross-disciplinary roles for an integrated approach
- Understand basic information for common mental health conditions: depressive disorder, bipolar disorder, anxiety, psychotic disorders, dementia, substance use disorder, and addiction
- Understand basic information for common childhood and adolescent mental health conditions: attention deficit hyperactivity disorder, autism, eating disorder, panic disorder, oppositional defiant disorder, and trauma
- Understand basic information for common chronic medical conditions: diabetes, heart failure, coronary artery disease, chronic obstructive pulmonary disease, asthma, and chronic kidney disease

For us to function as integrated case managers, we must be able to address all the patient's conditions. This requires that we have a general understanding of medical and behavioral conditions. For some, this may be uncomfortable or even a bit overwhelming as conditions that are unfamiliar to us will require our attention and intervention. We must be willing to learn about conditions less familiar so that we can support condition-changing treatment. In addition to broadening our knowledge base, we will have the support of an interdisciplinary team whose members may have experience that we lack. We draw upon our own experiences and consult with those who have knowledge in areas we do not in order to support our patients.

Cross-Disciplinary Roles

Integrated case management is a process in which a single case manager works with a patient to address all health concerns: medical, behavioral, social, and access to care. The assignment of a case manager should be based on the primary risk factors of the patient. The primary case manager should have expertise in those areas of risk. However, the expectation is that the primary case manager also works with the member in all areas that impact health, even if the case manager lacks specific experience with all the patient's conditions. In order to assist a patient regain health, we encourage case managers to become familiar with conditions less familiar. These may include the common conditions discussed in this chapter, or the patient may be challenged with less familiar conditions. Regardless, the case manager has a professional obligation to better understand the conditions, appropriate treatment, and associated challenges that may be faced.

To effectively function as an integrated case manager, it is not necessary to be an expert in the discipline with which we are less familiar. Case managers coming from a physical medicine background do not need to know every medication prescribed for every mental health condition, nor should the case manager coming from a behavioral health background need to know every medication prescribed for every physical health condition. Case managers assist patients in accessing needed care and services. That requires that we understand the direction in which to guide a patient and that we support the treatment prescribed by a physician. We do not recommend treatment. If we have a basic understanding of evidence-based treatments and have the support of a care team and physician advisor, we will be able to be effective in helping a patient move toward improved health. This basic understanding of illnesses and conditions provides us with the ability to assist a patient to remove barriers and access care that will result in illness improvement.

Guidelines for a basic understanding of illness:

- Recognize core signs and symptoms of the diagnosed condition(s)
- Know the common classes of medications used to treat a condition
- Know the resources needed to gain additional information about medications
- Understand the types of therapies that may be prescribed:
  - Psychotherapy: behavioral or cognitive
  - Physical therapy for orthopedic conditions
  - Occupational therapies for stroke, cerebral palsy, developmental delays, or other cognitive issues
  - Speech/language therapies for communication disorders
- Know how a patient should be monitored for his or her condition
- Know what constitutes a good response to treatment or what to look for if patient is not responding to treatment
- Know how to document progress or lack of progress
- Know when improvement should be expected once treatment has been initiated
- Know when and what to report if a patient is not making progress

Goals of Integrated Case Management

1. Have one primary case manager to address all of a patient's conditions, health concerns, social concerns, and barriers to improvement.

2. Case managers will familiarize themselves with the patient's conditions, prescribed treatment, and ability to follow the prescribed treatment plan.

3. Case managers will collaborate with the patient's clinicians to support the prescribed treatment.

4. Case managers will report to the clinicians any concerns related to complications, new symptoms, and the patient's ability to adhere to prescribed treatment.

5. Case managers will assist the patient in understanding his or her illness and how to eventually self-manage.

6. Case managers will assist the patient in removal of barriers preventing a return to health.

7. Case managers will encourage healthy behaviors and initiate conversations about change.

8. Case managers will report unnecessary or harmful care.

Case managers whose careers have focused primarily in one discipline or another may experience concern when asked to address a patient's issues in multiple domains. Supports need to be put in place so that all integrated case managers know where and how to get the information needed to be effective. We mentioned care teams in Chapter 2; an interdisciplinary care team should include:

- Medical case managers
- Behavioral case managers
- Nonclinical case manager extenders
- Pharmacy staff
- Community health workers/peer supports/community supports
- Medical director/physician advisor

The care team takes ownership of patients assigned. While there is one primary case manager working with a member, the team is there to aid and support. We have mentioned the professional responsibility of case managers to learn about unfamiliar conditions, but the experience of team members will also result in a widened knowledge base and comfort level. Interdisciplinary rounds are an excellent conduit for advice and recommendations as the team comes together to learn how patients are progressing. Rounds are a perfect venue for discussion of challenges as well as successes.

CASE STUDY

George has a long history of chronic obstructive pulmonary disease (COPD) and until recently managed his symptoms well. In the last 6 months, George has been in the emergency department (ED) four times and had a lengthy admission for pneumonia and respiratory distress. Callie, his case manager, reviewed his pharmacy utilization only to find that it appears George has not been filling his medications timely. When she talks with George, he is less than forthcoming about why he has not been filling his prescriptions. George tells Callie he just forgets to take his medicines sometimes and forgets to refill them. Callie is concerned because this is unusual for George. She brings George's case to interdisciplinary rounds. Callie's behavioral health (BH) team member Dan asks if Callie has screened George for depression. She has not, so Dan coaches Callie on how to begin the conversation to assess George for depression and recommends conducting the Patient Health Questionnaire (PHQ-9).

During Callie's next encounter with George, she begins to ask about "George" and does not talk about his COPD. She learns that George's grandson was recently killed while serving in Afghanistan. George admits he is devastated by the loss. Callie's work with George now takes a different focus and she works with her team to offer George services and resources that may assist with his grief and subsequent depression. There is an expectation that George will once again be able to self-manage his COPD, once his grief and depression are addressed. Repeated assessments using the PHQ-9 will provide data to demonstrate if strategies implemented to address George's grief and depression have been effective. ▪ ▪ ▪

How Case Managers Talk to Patients About Unhealthy Behaviors

Medical professionals are often uncomfortable asking questions about a patient's behavioral conditions, ability to cope, or unhealthy behaviors. We all know that "life happens" and the way we react to what comes our way differs from person to person. For the patient with complex conditions, the challenges of life can affect his or her ability to self-manage. Asking questions about a patient's emotional state are as important as understanding what physical symptoms the patient is experiencing. Overcoming this discomfort can be achieved by working with your behavioral health team members and colleagues and using scripting until the conversations become comfortable. The connection between physical concerns and emotional/behavioral responses leads to impairment in everyday functioning.

How Mental Health Professionals Address General Medical Disorders

Mental health professionals have traditionally avoided and been discouraged from addressing an individual's medical concerns. They have been taught that the mind and body are not connected; this is contrary to the beliefs of many ancient cultures and to holistic practice. Avoidance of addressing physical concerns along with behavioral concerns was thought to result in a transference of behaviors to physical symptoms. The lack of confidence in addressing medical concerns also leads to avoidance. For mental health professionals to become effective integrated case managers, they must be willing to address medical issues.

Regardless of your primary discipline, much can be learned through conversation and use of open-ended questions. Through conversation, and not interrogation, much can be learned from the patient about his or her health, feelings, concerns, and hopes. These conversations also build trust with the patient and promote engagement.

Suggested Assessment Questions for Both Physical and Behavioral Case Managers

- General life questions
  - "Hello Ms./Mr. _____, my name is _____ and I am a nurse/social worker from your benefit plan _____. I'm reaching out as it appears you have been having some health problems lately. I would very much like to assist you in any way needed. Would it be alright if I ask you a few questions?"
  - "Can you tell me what health problems concern you the most?"
  - "How has _____ affected your everyday life?"

- Physical health
  - "How have you been managing your _____?"
  - "What worries you the most right now?"
  - "Can you tell me what you see are challenges to managing your _____?"
  - "How often do you see your doctor?"
- Emotional health
  - "How does your health affect you emotionally?"
  - "Are you feeling worried, anxious, sad?"
  - "How many days do you feel worried, anxious, sad?"
  - "Do you have trouble remembering things?"
  - "If so, what things are hard to remember?"
- Relationships with providers
  - "Whom do you see for your health problems?"
  - "Do you feel as though you have a good relationship with Dr. _____?"
- Access to care
  - "Are you able to get appointments with your doctor when needed?"
  - "If not, what do you see as the problem?"
  - "When you have appointments, do you have any problems getting there?"
  - "Do your health benefits adequately cover the care you need?" (prescriptions, co-pays)
- Social issues
  - "Who is available to help you when you need it?"
  - "Do you feel safe where you live?"
  - "If no, what are your safety concerns?"
  - "Do you have a job?" (includes full-time homemaker; for children, school)
  - "Are you able to meet your financial obligations?"
  - "If no, what financial challenges do you face?"

- Additional information
  - "Right now, what is your greatest concern?"
  - "What would you like to work on?"
  - "What things did I not ask that you would like for me to know?"

Important Issues Related to Medical and Mental Health Care

When examining the considerations that professionals from either the medical or mental health disciplines require, there are some significant differences, especially for mental health. Rarely is treatment for medical conditions forced. The exception is the presence of communicable diseases. Individuals with severe psychiatric illness may be examined for competency or involuntary commitment via court-ordered action. Forced admission or detention occurs when an individual's judgment is impaired to the point of risk, or he or she is a physical threat to self or others. Examples of conditions that can escalate these risks are dementia, substance abuse, eating disorders, or psychosis. Case managers are typically not involved in the legal process but should understand the process. The role of the case manager in these situations is to provide support to the patient and his or her support system, and to assist in the coordination of care and services at the conclusion of the commitment or detention. Laws related to competency and commitment vary from state to state, and case managers must familiarize themselves with the process in their local jurisdictions.

Patients who verbalize suicidal or homicidal thoughts are at significant risk. Case managers from a medical background may find this expression frightening. When a patient expresses such thoughts, you as a case manager must be proactive and determine the level of intent. There are ways to determine how to escalate your intervention. Have discussions with your behavioral health team members. Ask them to share some real-life experiences with you and ask that they share how they have handled such crises.

Understanding Mental Health and Behavioral Disorders

The terms "mental" and "behavioral" are often used interchangeably but it is important to understand that there is a difference between mental/psychiatric illness and behavioral disorder. Mental disorders have been defined by a variety of concepts like "distress," "irrationality," and "inflexibility," just to name a few (Stein, Phillips, Bolton, & Fulford, 2010). Debate continues as to how best to define these conditions but according to *DSM-5*, the more modern, philosophical and neuroscientific views recommend the term "psychiatric disorder" versus "mental disorder" (Stein et al., 2010). The term "mental" seems to limit the focus and implies the mind and brain are separate, distinct realms. So until there can be some consensus, the interim term is "mental/psychiatric disorder" (Stein et al., 2010).

It is equally important to realize that behavior plays a role in both mental/psychiatric disorders and behavioral disorders. Mental/psychiatric disorders affect mood, thinking, behavior, and impairment of mental faculties. Mental/psychiatric disorders may also manifest involuntary signs and symptoms. Individuals may experience disabilities that impact their ability to perform daily functions (Stein et al., 2010).

Behavioral conditions are not psychiatric in origin; however, behaviors may affect the individual's ability to function. Typically, behavioral disorders are a dysfunction in behavior and include a behavior that can be controlled, such as anorexia nervosa, substance use disorders, or posttraumatic stress disorder (Stein et al., 2010).

General Procedures for Handling Suicidal Thoughts/Expressions

The patient expressing thoughts of self-harm requires the case manager to listen carefully and clarify intent. Be aware of risk factors that can lead to thoughts and plans for self-harm: depression, drug/alcohol intoxication, an acute crisis, history of prior suicide attempts, and worsening life circumstances.

Level 1: The patient expresses a lack of fear of death; does not want to live ("Life just doesn't seem worth living.").

Level 2: The patient expresses active thoughts of harming self ("I want to kill myself.").

Level 3: The patient expresses a method for self-harm, but not a plan ("I want to shoot myself.").

Level 4: The patient expresses a method and a plan for self-harm ("I have a gun and I'm going to shoot myself"; "I won't be here tomorrow.").

Interventions based on the level of risk

Level 1:   Tell the patient you are going to connect them with help. Contact the treating psychiatrist or therapist to schedule an emergent appointment. Keep the patient on the phone if possible and ask a team member to contact the provider for the appointment.

Levels 2–4: Directly transfer the patient to a crisis intervention service. If the patient refuses, call 911. If the member reports an imminent attempt, call 911 to dispatch emergency responders.

General Procedures for Handling Homicidal Thoughts/Expressions

- Listen to the patient carefully and clarify what you have heard.
- Strongly encourage the patient to contact his or her mental health provider; if unwilling, contact the provider to facilitate an emergent appointment or ask a team member to contact the provider while you stay on the phone with the patient.
- Try to maintain your relationship with the member, how you are here to help, but do not get caught up in the patient's disputes with others.
- Discuss the situation with your medical director or physician advisor.
- If the patient verbalizes a direct threat to a specific individual, you have an obligation to contact and warn that individual and to notify law enforcement.

Addressing Medical Emergencies

Case managers who do not come from a medical background also need to know what to do in a medical emergency. Knowing what to do in every emergency is not feasible, but with medical emergencies the best strategy is common sense. Case managers must always err on the side of caution, keeping the patient's safety as the priority. That may mean conducting a three-way call with the treating physician, sending the patient to the ED, and calling emergency responders yourself. Conditions that indicate a medical emergency may be occurring include, but are not limited to, the following:

- Chest pain
- Shortness of breath
- Severe diaphoresis (perspiring, feeling clammy)
- Severe weakness
- Any combination of these conditions
- Gastrointestinal bleeding (vomiting blood or dark vomit, bleeding from the rectum)
- Severe headache
- Weakness on one side of the body
- Confusion
- Loss of speech or vision

Pediatric Emergencies

Reacting to pediatric medical or behavioral emergencies is subject to the same guidelines as adults. Case managers working with pediatric populations are also challenged with knowing and understanding local legislation as it pertains to the age of consent. Depending on your local jurisdiction, adolescents may have a voice in the consent to release information or share protected health information. We must also be aware of legislation related to the reporting of child abuse and neglect; laws may differ from state to state. Ultimately, the child's safety and well-being must be the priority and we must always act in that child's best interest.

Child abuse and neglect are generally defined as any type of cruel act inflicted on a child including physical harm, emotional abuse, neglect in care like isolation or withholding food, or sexual abuse and exploitation. Known or suspected child abuse and neglect are subject to mandatory reporting. Failure to report known or suspected abuse and neglect to protective agencies can be criminally prosecuted. If you as the case manager are unsure of the presence of abuse and neglect, consult your supervisor or medical director. Again, the welfare and safety of the child is paramount.

Common Medical Conditions

Let us examine some of the common medical mental/psychiatric and behavioral conditions (see Tables 6.1–6.12). The content included, developed from multiple sources, should guide your information search for any unfamiliar condition (American Psychological Association, n.d.; National Alliance on Mental Illness [NAMI], n.d.; Godara, Hirbe, Nassif, Otepka, & Rosenstock, 2014).

TABLE 6.1 Diabetes Mellitus

Types of diabetes	Type I; Type II; Gestational
Epidemiology	This is the most common form of diabetes, the one with which most are familiar. Diabetes insipidus is a different condition. It is much less common and treated differently. • Diabetes is an endocrine disorder in which insulin, the hormone that transfers sugar from the blood to cells (for energy) during food digestion, is either not produced by the pancreas or the insulin that is produced is of poor quality. • In type I diabetes, the pancreas produces little to no insulin so it must be replaced: insulin injections or continuous infusion via a pump. Type I diabetes can be diagnosed in childhood or adulthood. • In type II diabetes, the pancreas ineffectively produces insulin; either it is not strong enough to achieve its function, or it is ineffectively used by the body. • Gestational diabetes is the development of diabetes during pregnancy. Babies are often larger than normal and may have hypoglycemia after birth. The diabetes often dissipates in the mother after pregnancy but leaves her at risk of developing diabetes later in life.
Signs and symptoms of diabetes	• Increased thirst • Frequent urination • Weight loss • Poorly healing wounds • Frequent infections
Complications of poor control	• Elevated blood glucose (hyperglycemia) • Hyperglycemia over time will damage eyes, kidneys, and nerves • Heart disease • Peripheral vascular disease: amputations, poorly healing wounds Regardless of the type of diabetes, untreated hyperglycemia will result in these conditions, especially over time. Often the most damaging is severe fluctuations in high versus low blood sugar.

(continued)

TABLE 6.1 Diabetes Mellitus (*continued*)

Tests to measure glucose (blood sugar)	• Hemoglobin A1c • Urine (sugar and ketones) • FBS • Self-monitoring The hemoglobin A1c and a FBS >200 are often the tests done to diagnose diabetes. The HgbA1c is also repeated 2–4 times per year to measure diabetes control. The test provides an average over a 3-month period. According to the American Diabetes Association, the target HgbA1c is <7%. If a member is spilling sugar or ketones in the urine, diabetes is not controlled. Spilling sugar indicates hyperglycemia, ketones indicate hypoglycemia. A FBS is often the first test done to screen for diabetes. A FBS >200 warrants additional testing. Once diagnosed, the member can self-monitor using a finger stick to collect a small amount of blood and test with a glucometer.
Diabetes management: type I	• Diet • Exercise • Medication Regardless of the type of diabetes, these are the standard treatment approaches. In type II it is possible for members to manage their diabetes with diet and exercise alone! • Insulin replacement • Regular monitoring of blood sugar • Dietary modifications: balance of carbohydrates and proteins • Exercise • Regular monitoring of blood sugar, kidney function, blood pressure, lipids, vision, skin • Physician follow-up: PCP quarterly, endocrinologist at least annually unless complications are present; then increased visits to an endocrinologist may be necessary

Diabetes management: type II	Individuals with type II diabetes will not always require medication; they can be managed by diet and exercise alone in some cases. That said, they may also require insulin replacement in addition to oral diabetic medications to better regulate blood sugar.
	• Dietary modifications: balance of carbohydrates and proteins
	• Exercise
	• Medication
	  ■ Sulfonylureas stimulate the pancreas to release more insulin, i.e., glipizide
	  ■ Biquanides: decrease the amount of sugar produced by the liver; i.e., metformin
	  ■ Meglitinides stimulate the pancreas to release more insulin, i.e., repaglinide

(continued)

TABLE 6.1 Diabetes Mellitus (*continued*)

	■ Thiazolidinediones boost insulin's ability to reduce glucose, i.e., Avandia ■ DPP-4 inhibitors reduce serum glucose without causing hypoglycemia, i.e., Januvia ■ SGLT2 inhibitors absorb glucose in the kidney, i.e., Invokana ■ Long-acting insulin, i.e., Levemir ■ Intermediate-acting insulin, i.e., Humulin-N ■ Short-acting insulin, i.e., Humulin-R ■ Rapid-acting insulin, i.e., Novolog • Regular monitoring of blood sugar based on physician orders • Physician follow-up: PCP quarterly, endocrinologist if complications are present
Diabetes surveillance	• Hemoglobin A1c: 2–4 times per year • Self-monitoring of glucose: per MD orders • Annual exams: eye, kidney, serum cholesterol, blood pressure if no hypertension
Resources	• American Diabetes Association (www.diabetes.org) • National Libraries of Medicine (www.nlm.nih.gov/medline/diabetes)

DPP-4, dipeptidyl peptidase-4; FBS, fasting blood sugar; SGLT2, sodium-glucose co-transporter 2.
Source: Godara, Hirbe, Nassif, Otepka, & Rosenstock (2014).

TABLE 6.2 Heart Disease

Types of heart disease	• Cardiovascular disease • Heart failure Heart disease is an overarching term that can include multiple conditions and disorders from congenital causes to lifestyle-induced. For the purposes of this presentation, we discuss two of the most common conditions: CAD and CHF.
Epidemiology: cardiovascular disease/CAD	The arteries that supply the heart muscle become narrowed and/ or hardened. This occurs as a result of cholesterol and other forms of plaque lining the artery walls. The buildup itself is called "atherosclerosis." As the arteries continue to narrow from the buildup, the heart muscle is deprived of oxygenated blood. This reduced blood flow or "starved" heart muscle results in chest pain or angina. When pieces of the plaque are large enough to block an artery, or the artery becomes completely occluded, a heart attack or MI can occur. The loss of oxygen to the heart muscle results in permanent damage.

(*continued*)

TABLE 6.2 Heart Disease (*continued*)

	The pain felt before and during, and the resulting death of the muscle is a heart attack. Over time CAD weakens the heart muscle and can cause arrhythmias and heart failure. • Leading cause of death in men and women • Narrowed or "clogged" arteries • Can lead to heart attack **Normal Artery**　　**Narrowing of Artery** Lipid deposit of plaque Coronary Artery Disease Medical gallery of Blausen Medical 2014. WikiJournal of Medicine 1 (2).
Signs and symptoms of cardiovascular disease	• Chest pain or chest discomfort 　■ Chest pressure 　■ "Squeezing" sensation in the chest 　■ Pain in shoulders, arms, neck, jaw 　■ Indigestion 　■ Pain worsens with activity, lessens with rest • Shortness of breath • No symptoms 　■ Some individuals will have no symptoms, or will not report symptoms until they actually have a heart attack
Risk factors	• Family history • Elevated lipids: cholesterol, triglycerides • Smoking • HTN • Insulin resistance • Diabetes • Obesity • Lack of physical activity • Sleep apnea The risk factors can be extensive. Family history is the most important to assess: we cannot change our genetic makeup; so then it becomes even more important to reduce the other risk factors listed. For those who do not know, cholesterol and triglycerides are lipids that contribute to plaque or narrowing of arteries. Insulin resistance is

(continued)

TABLE 6.2 Heart Disease (*continued*)

	often the condition that occurs prior to a diagnosis of diabetes, and sleep apnea is a condition whereby periods of apnea, or lack of breath during sleep, reduce oxygen levels that can then lead to HTN.
Tests to diagnose cardiovascular disease	<ul><li>EKG<ul><li>EKG: can show damage to the heart muscle from a previous or current MI</li></ul></li><li>Stress test<ul><li>Exercise is used to make the heart work hard and beat fast; when this happens, the heart needs more blood and oxygen— if arteries are occluded or narrowed, the test shows abnormal changes in the heart rhythm and blood pressure, which then may cause shortness of breath and chest pain.</li></ul></li><li>Echocardiogram<ul><li>Sound waves are used to produce images of the heart. The function of the heart is examined to see if it is pumping properly.</li></ul></li><li>Cardiac catheterization (or angiogram)<ul><li>This is an interventional procedure in which a dye is injected into the femoral artery (typically) using a long, thin catheter. The dye and use of the catheter help to visualize any blockages in the coronary arteries.</li></ul></li></ul> 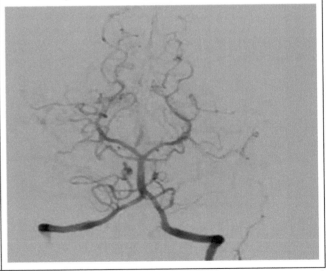

Copyright © Wikimedia, Lipothymia.

(continued)

TABLE 6.2 Heart Disease (*continued*)

Treatment of cardiovascular disease	• Conservative measures ▪ Quit smoking ▪ Eat a healthy diet ▪ Exercise regularly ▪ Lose any excess weight ▪ Reduce stress • Medications ▪ Cholesterol modifiers ▪ ASA: aspirin to reduce clotting ▪ Nitroglycerin ▪ Beta-blockers ▪ ACE inhibitor or ARBs • Surgical interventions ▪ Angioplasty and stent placement (PCR) ▪ CABG PCR or percutaneous coronary revascularization/PCI is the result of angioplasty with stent placement. A catheter is inserted into a narrowed artery, a wire with a deflated balloon is passed through the catheter and then inflated. The balloon compresses plaque deposits and the vessel is opened. A small mesh tube, or stent, may be placed and left in the vessel to maintain patency. The stents are actually medicated and release medication to help keep the vessel from re-occluding.
Epidemiology: heart failure	• CHF • Right-sided heart failure • Left-sided heart failure Heart failure is a condition in which the heart is unable to pump enough blood to meet the body's needs. Heart failure can occur on one or both sides of the heart. Heart failure means the heart is weakened. 　Because the heart is weakened from CAD, HTN, diabetes, or other causes such as infection or congenital anomaly, it cannot pump efficiently or effectively. This results in blood and fluid backing up into the lungs causing swelling (edema) in the feet, ankles, legs, or abdomen; fatigue; and shortness of breath. Heart failure is more common in people over the age of 65, African Americans, those who are overweight, and those who have already had a heart attack. 　There is no cure for heart failure, but there are treatment options that can result in a longer, more active life.

(continued)

TABLE 6.2 Heart Disease (*continued*)

Signs and symptoms of heart failure	• Shortness of breath • Fatigue • Edema All of these symptoms occur as a result of fluid backup in the body. As the heart grows weaker, the symptoms get worse.
Risk factors of heart failure	• Past medical history of heart disease (CAD) • Family history of heart failure • History of a heart attack Poorly managed CAD and HTN will result in weaker heart function resulting in heart failure. History of a heart attack or family history of heart failure also increase risks.

Tests to diagnose heart failure	• Physical exam
	• EKG
	• Chest x-ray
	• BNP
	• Echocardiogram
	  ■ Upon physical exam, the physician will listen to heart and breath sounds, looking for irregular rhythm or decreased breath sounds. The physician will also examine the extremities to evaluate for any edema.
	  ■ An EKG is done to evaluate the possibility of an arrhythmia.
	  ■ Chest x-ray will visualize any fluid backup in the lungs.
	  ■ BNP is a hormone that will be increased in heart failure.
	  ■ The echo will review the size and action of the heart valves, and will look to see if blood flow is decreased.

Goals of treatment	• Treat underlying conditions (CAD, HTN, DM) • Decrease signs and symptoms • Prevent further progression • Improve quality of life and life expectancy Early diagnosis and treatment help people with heart failure to live longer, more active lives. Treatment depends on the severity of the failure.
Conservative treatment options	• Quit smoking • Healthy diet • Fluid intake • Weight loss • Physician-advised activity level Changes in habits or choices like smoking, eating a healthy diet, modifying fluid intake as prescribed, losing weight, following a physician-prescribed activity level can result in decreased heart failure symptoms.

(continued)

TABLE 6.2 Heart Disease (*continued*)

Medications	Some of the medications were reviewed with CAD: • Diuretics are used to remove excess fluid through the kidneys. • Aldosterone antagonists trigger the excretion of sodium and fluid through the kidneys; this results in a decrease of blood volume which will decrease the work of the heart. • Isosorbide/hydralazine relaxes blood vessels to decrease the work of the heart. • Digoxin helps the heart beat more effectively. • Oxygen is used in advanced disease and replaces oxygen not made available by a weakened heart.
Surgical/procedural interventions	• Implantable defibrillator (also known as cardiac resynchronization therapy) • Pacemaker • LVAD • Heart transplant For more serious heart failure, more aggressive therapies are required. Implantable devises may be required to help the heartbeat. • For poor contractility, a pacemaker will help the heart beat regularly. • If there is a threat that the heart could stop beating, an implantable defibrillator will jumpstart the heart. • When the heart can literally not pump enough blood to sustain life, the LVAD will be implanted to take over and assist the heart. While this device can be used long term, you typically see it before a transplant. • A heart transplant is a life-saving intervention and listing will occur when there is little or no hope that other treatments can sustain life indefinitely.
Important self-care	• Making and keeping regular appointments with physicians • Reporting weight gain over short periods of time, e.g., ≥3 lbs in 24 hours • Controlling other conditions • Avoiding respiratory infections These areas are where the case manager can have the most impact. These interventions require adherence on the part of the member. Promoting that adherence and self-care can make all the difference in how well the member's heart failure is managed.
Resources	• American Heart Association (www.heart.org)

ACE, angiotensin-converting enzyme; ARBs, angiotensin II retention blockers; ASA, acetylsalicylic acid (aspirin); BNP, brain natriuretic peptide; CABG, coronary artery bypass graft; CAD, coronary artery disease; CHF, congestive heart failure; DM, diabetes mellitus; HTN, hypertension; LVAD, left ventricular assist device; MI, myocardial infarction; PCI, percutaneous coronary intervention.
Source: Godara, Hirbe, Nassif, Otepka, & Rosenstock (2014).

TABLE 6.3 Kidney Disease

Types of kidney disease	• CKD • Kidney failure Our kidneys, located in the mid to low back, are about the size of our fist. Their role is to filter waste and excess fluid from the blood; this results in urine which is then excreted. This filtering process also helps keep the body's chemical balance, helps control blood pressure, and makes hormones.
Etiology of kidney disease	CKD means that one or both kidneys are damaged and cannot filter the wastes from the blood. Diabetes and high blood pressure are known to damage kidneys if they are not properly controlled. Over time, if CKD is not controlled, the kidneys will fail. Once this happens, dialysis or kidney transplant is required.
Signs and symptoms of kidney disease	• Fatigue • Weakness • Loss of appetite • Insomnia • Unable to think clearly • Swelling in feet and ankles Unfortunately, most people do not notice symptoms when the disease is in its early stages. However, as the disease progresses, one can expect these symptoms.
Risk factors	• Congenital conditions • Diabetes • High blood pressure • Heart disease • Chronic urinary tract infections • Urinary blockages Conditions whereby there is compromise to blood flow, like DB, HTN, and heart disease, are likely the most common causes of kidney disease. Chronic infections and blockages also result in destruction of the kidneys which results in failure.
Tests to diagnose and monitor kidney disease	• Blood pressure monitoring • Urine albumin • Serum creatinine Routine screening for kidney disease is not recommended. If a member has chronic or poorly controlled diabetes, hypertension, and/or heart disease, it would be important for the physician to order these tests.

(continued)

TABLE 6.3 Kidney Disease (*continued*)

Goals of treatment	• Prevent progression of kidney disease to kidney failure Kidney disease is usually rated by stages. Stages 4 and 5 indicate dialysis or perhaps even transplant is indicated.
Management of kidney disease	• Control blood pressure and diabetes • Quit smoking • Eat less protein • Schedule and keep regular appointments • Medication • Dialysis • Kidney transplant While kidney failure may or may not be completely preventable once advanced disease is present, efforts can continue to slow the progression.
Resources	MedlinePlus (www.nlm.nih.gov/medlineplus/chronickidneydisease.html)

CKD, chronic kidney disease; HTN, hypertension.

TABLE 6.4 Asthma

Epidemiology	Asthma is a chronic disease characterized by acute exacerbations caused by bronchial tube swelling and increased production of mucous. Unlike COPD, the individual with asthma will have symptom-free periods.
Symptoms of asthma	• Shortness of breath • Chest tightness • Chronic coughing • Wheezing • Trouble sleeping linked to coughing and/or wheezing
Risk factors	• Allergens • Upper respiratory infection • Occupational exposures related to pollutants, dust, particulates • Smoke (of any kind) • Emotional distress • Exercise intolerance • Medications (NSAIDs, ASA)
Tests to diagnose asthma	None—asthma is diagnosed based on the first exacerbation

(continued)

TABLE 6.4 Asthma (*continued*)

Management of asthma	<ul><li>Education<ul><li>How to prevent exacerbations</li><li>What triggers exacerbations</li></ul></li><li>Avoid asthma triggers<ul><li>Control allergies</li></ul></li><li>Annual flu vaccination</li><li>Improving coping skills</li><li>Asthma action plan<ul><li>What to do when symptoms start</li><li>When to go to the ED</li></ul></li><li>Adherence with physician follow-up and prescribed treatment</li><li>Medications<ul><li>Short-acting bronchodilators—Albuterol</li><li>Long-acting bronchodilators</li><li>Inhaled corticosteroids</li></ul></li></ul>
Resources	Asthma and Allergy Foundation of America (www.aafa.org)

ASA, acetylsalicylic acid (aspirin); COPD, chronic obstructive pulmonary disease; ED, emergency department; NSAIDs, non-steroidal anti-inflammatory drugs.

TABLE 6.5 Chronic Obstructive Pulmonary Disease

Epidemiology	COPD is a group of chronic inflammatory lung diseases characterized by obstructed airflow due to alveolar damage. The most common types are emphysema, chronic bronchitis, and refractory asthma. The causes of COPD include tobacco smoking, inhalation of pollutants such as smoke, fumes, chemicals, and dust.
Signs and symptoms of COPD	<ul><li>Shortness of breath</li><li>Wheezing</li><li>Chest tightness</li><li>Clearing throat of excess mucous</li><li>Chronic cough with or without mucous</li><li>Cyanosis of lips or fingertips</li><li>Frequent respiratory infections</li><li>Lack of energy</li><li>Unintended weight loss</li><li>Swelling of lower extremities</li></ul>
Risk factors	<ul><li>Tobacco smoking</li><li>Inhalation of occupational pollutants</li></ul>

(continued)

TABLE 6.5 Chronic Obstructive Pulmonary Disease (*continued*)

Tests to diagnose COPD	• Lung function tests • Chest x-ray • CT scan of chest • Arterial blood gases (typically done only in the acute care setting)

Management of COPD	• Stop smoking tobacco
	• Medications
	  ■ Short-acting bronchodilators
	  ■ Long-acting bronchodilators
	  ■ Inhaled corticosteroids
	  ■ Combination inhalers (bronchodilators + steroids)
	  ■ Oral steroids
	  ■ Theophylline
	  ■ Antibiotics
	  ■ Phosphodiesterase-4 inhibitors
	• Pulmonary rehabilitation
	  ■ Improve lung function
	  ■ Improve exercise/activity tolerance
	• Oxygen therapy
	  ■ When lung function has deteriorated to the point of ineffective oxygenation for the body

Resources	COPD Foundation (www.copdfoundation.org)

COPD, chronic obstructive pulmonary disease.

Common Mental Health Conditions

TABLE 6.6 Anxiety Disorders

Epidemiology	Anxiety disorders are a group of disorders characterized by excessive anxiety or worry that persists for lengthy periods (months or *longer*). Types of anxiety disorders: • Generalized anxiety disorder • Panic disorder • Agoraphobia • Anxiety due to a medical condition • Selective mutism • Substance *use–induced* anxiety • Specific phobias • Unspecified anxiety disorder

(continued)

TABLE 6.6 Anxiety Disorders (*continued*)

Signs and symptoms of anxiety disorders	• Feeling nervous, tense, restless • Sense of impending doom, danger, or panic • Increased heart rate • Sweating or trembling • Hyperventilation • Feeling weak or tired • Difficulty concentrating or thinking about anything other than the current worry • Difficulty sleeping • Gastrointestinal problems • Avoiding things that trigger anxiety • Difficulty controlling worry
Risk factors for developing anxiety disorders	• Shyness or behavioral inhibition in childhood • Being female • Limited economic resources • Exposures to stressful life events in childhood or adulthood • Family history

Management of anxiety disorders	• Therapy
	  ■ Cognitive behavioral therapy
	• Medications
	  ■ Benzodiazepines
	  ■ Antidepressants
	    – SSRI
	    – SNRI
	  ■ Tricyclic antidepressants
	  ■ Mild tranquilizer
	  ■ Anticonvulsants
	  ■ Beta-blockers

Resources	American Psychological Association (www.apa.org)

SNRI, serotonin–norepinephrine reuptake inhibitor; SSRI, selective serotonin reuptake inhibitor.

TABLE 6.7 Depressive Disorders

Epidemiology	Depressive disorders are a group of mood disorders characterized by persistent feelings of sadness and loss of interest. Included in this group are: • Major depression • Situational depression • Bipolar disorder • Psychotic depression • Postpartum depression • Persistent depressive disorder • SAD • PMDD

(*continued*)

TABLE 6.7 Depressive Disorders (*continued*)

	The causes of depression can be organic or environmental: • Family history • Genetic factors • Brain chemistry • Hormones • Life events
Signs and symptoms of depression	• Feelings of sadness, tearfulness, emptiness, hopelessness • Angry outbursts • Loss of interest or pleasure • Sleep disturbances • Anxiety, restlessness, or agitation • Slowed thinking or movement • Difficulty thinking or concentrating • Unexplained physical problems • Frequent or recurrent thoughts of death or suicide • Changes in appetite • Lack of energy
Complications of depression	• Weight gain or obesity • Pain and physical illness • Alcohol or substance misuse • Anxiety • Panic disorder • Social isolation • Difficulty with current relationships • Self-mutilation • Premature death • Suicidal feelings or attempts

Management of depression	• Therapy
	  ■ Cognitive behavioral therapy
	• Antidepressants
	  ■ SSRI
	  ■ SNRI
	• Tricyclic antidepressants
	• ECT
	Talking therapies should be the first line of treatment with medication for support. Conditions like bipolar disorder will almost always require medication. ECT is an option when response to therapy and medication has been ineffective.

Resources	National Alliance on Mental Illness (www.nami.org) American Psychological Association (www.apa.org)

ECT, electroconvulsive therapy; PMDD, premenstrual dysphoric disorder; SAD, seasonal affective disorder; SNRI, serotonin–norepinephrine reuptake inhibitor; SSRI, selective serotonin reuptake inhibitor.

TABLE 6.8 Psychotic Disorders

Epidemiology	Psychotic disorders are a group of serious mental illnesses characterized by the individual losing touch with reality and experiencing a range of symptoms including hallucinations and delusions. The conditions listed are forms of SMI and SPMI. Causes of psychotic disorders are linked to birth complications, family history use of psychoactive medications, and even immune system activation. Types of psychotic disorders: • Schizophrenia • Bipolar disorder • Schizotypal personality disorder • Catatonia • Delusional disorder • Substance or medication-induced psychotic disorder
Signs and symptoms of psychotic disorders	• Delusions and hallucinations • Disorganized thinking and speech • Abnormal movements • Difficulty sleeping • Irritability or depressed mood • Lack of motivation
Complications of psychotic disorders	• Suicidal thoughts or attempts • Self-harm/injury • Anxiety disorders and obsessive-compulsive disorder • Depression • Substance use • Inability to work or attend school • Social isolation • Homelessness • Legal and financial problems • Being victimized or traumatized
Management of psychotic disorders	These treatment options are often used in combination. Without management, individuals with serious mental illness are at a high risk of hospitalization. • Medication ▪ Antipsychotics (multiple classifications) ▪ Combination psychotherapeutic agents • Cognitive behavioral therapies • ECT • Confinement for management
Resources	• American Psychological Association (www.apa.org) • National Alliance on Mental Illness (www.nami.org)

ECT, electroconvulsive therapy; SMI, serious mental illness; SPMI, serious and persistent mental illness.

TABLE 6.9 Substance Use

Epidemiology	Substance use disorders are classified as the use of one or more substances to the extent to which an individual is clinically and functionally impaired. Addiction is included in this description. Substance use may occur as a result of environmental factors, life events, and genetic predisposition. Tobacco use is included as an addiction.
Risk factors for substance use	• Family history of addiction • Being male • Having another mental disorder • Peer pressure • Lack of family involvement or support • Anxiety, depression, and loneliness • Taking highly addictive prescription medications
Signs and symptoms of substance use	• Intense urges for the substance of choice • Focusing more time and energy on obtaining the substance • Withdrawal and tolerance • Behavioral changes • Changes in spending habits • Inability to meet obligations and responsibilities • Reckless behavior
Complications of substance use	• Move to multiple types of substances • Risk of contracting infectious disease • Accidents while under the influence • Suicide • Relationship problems • Work or school issues • Legal and financial problems • Short-term or long-term physical health problems

Management of substance use	• Detoxification
	  ■ Supervision usually required
	• Counseling
	• Self-help groups
	  ■ Alcoholics Anonymous
	  ■ Narcotics Anonymous

Resources	• American Psychological Association (www.apa.org) • National Alliance on Mental Illness (www.nami.org)

TABLE 6.10 Attention Deficit Hyperactivity Disorder

Epidemiology	ADHD is a condition which is characterized by inattention, hyperactivity, and impulsivity. ADHD is most commonly diagnosed in young people, according to the CDC. An estimated 9% of children between ages 3 and 17 have ADHD. While ADHD is usually diagnosed in childhood, it does not only affect children. An estimated 4% of adults have ADHD. Causes of ADHD are believed to be genetic and environmental. ADHD does seem to run in families. Exposure to cigarette smoking and alcohol during pregnancy and lead exposure during childhood are contributors.
Signs and symptoms of ADHD	Individuals with ADHD have difficulty controlling the following symptoms and the duration is greater than 6 months. Signs of inattention: • Becoming easily distracted and jumping from activity to activity • Becoming bored with a task quickly • Difficulty focusing attention or completing a single task or activity • Trouble completing or turning in homework assignments • Losing things such as school supplies or toys • Not listening or paying attention when spoken to • Daydreaming or wandering with lack of motivation • Difficulty processing information quickly • Struggling to follow directions Signs of hyperactivity: • Fidgeting and squirming, having trouble sitting still • Non-stop talking • Touching or playing with everything • Difficulty doing quiet tasks or activities Signs of impulsivity: • Impatience • Acting without regard for consequences, blurting things out • Difficulty taking turns, waiting or sharing • Interrupting others
Diagnostic tests for ADHD	ADHD occurs in both children and adults, but is most often and diagnosed in childhood. Getting a diagnosis for ADHD can sometimes be difficult because the symptoms of ADHD are similar to typical behavior in most young children. Teachers are often the first to notice ADHD symptoms because they see children in a learning environment with peers every day. There is no one single test that can diagnose a child with ADHD, so meet with a doctor or mental health professional to gather all the necessary information to make a diagnosis. The goal is to rule out any outside causes for symptoms, such as environmental changes, difficulty in school, medical problems, and ensure that a child is otherwise healthy.

(continued)

TABLE 6.10 Attention Deficit Hyperactivity Disorder (*continued*)

Complications of ADHD	Children with ADHD often have other conditions that make management difficult. These include: • Learning disability • Oppositional defiant disorder • Conduct disorders: disruptive, destructive, or violent behaviors • Depression • Anxiety • Obsessive-compulsive disorder • Substance use • Bipolar disorder • Tourette's syndrome • Sleep disorders • Bed-wetting
Management of ADHD	• Behavioral therapies • Alternative therapies conducted by schools and employers ▪ Educational support and assistance ▪ Self-management programs • Medications ▪ Stimulants ▪ Non-stimulants ▪ Antidepressants

ADHD, attention deficit hyperactivity disorder; CDC, Centers for Disease Control and Prevention.

TABLE 6.11 Autism

Epidemiology	• ASD is a developmental disorder that affects a person's ability to socialize and communicate with others. ASD can also result in restricted, repetitive patterns of behavior, interests, or activities. The term "spectrum" refers to the wide range of symptoms, skills, and levels of impairment or disability that people with ASD can display. Some people are mildly impaired by their symptoms, while others are severely disabled. The prevalence rate for ASD is 1 in 68 children and rising. Boys are 4 times more likely than girls to develop autism. ASD crosses racial, ethnic, and social backgrounds equally. Awareness of this disorder and improved screening methods have contributed to the increase in diagnoses in recent years. There is no clear cause of autism. Scientists believe there may be several causes: • Genetics: If one child in a family has ASD, another sibling is more likely to develop it too. Likewise, identical twins are highly likely to both develop autism if it is present. Relatives of children with autism show minor signs of communication difficulties. Scans reveal that people on the autism spectrum have certain abnormalities of the brain's structure and chemical function.

(continued)

TABLE 6.11 Autism (*continued*)

	• Environment: Scientists are currently researching many environmental factors that are thought to play a role in contributing to ASD. Many prenatal factors may contribute to a child's development, such as a mother's health. Other postnatal factors may affect development as well. Despite many claims that have been highlighted by the media, strong evidence has been shown that vaccines do not cause autism.
Diagnostic tests for autism	There is no medical test that can determine the possibility of developing autism. Specialists make the diagnosis after screening for social deficits, communication problems, and repetitive or restricted behavior. Diagnosing autism is often a two-stage process. The first stage involves general developmental screening during well-child checkups with a pediatrician. Children who show some developmental problems are referred for more evaluation. The second stage involves a thorough evaluation by a team of doctors and other health professionals with a wide range of specialties. At this stage, a child may be diagnosed as having autism or another developmental disorder. Typically, children with ASD can be reliably diagnosed by age 2, though some may not be diagnosed until they are older. Screening tools that may be used by health care professionals to diagnose autism: • M-CHAT: Modified Checklist for Autism in Toddlers • STAT: Screening Tool for Autism in Two-year-olds • SCQ: Social Communication Questionnaire • CSBS: Communication and Symbolic Behavior Scales
Signs and symptoms of autism	Symptoms of autism fall on a continuum. This means that the learning, thinking, and problem-solving abilities of children with ASD can range from gifted to severely challenged. Some children with ASD need a lot of help in their daily lives. With a thorough evaluation, doctors can make a diagnosis to help find the best treatment plan for the child. • Delay in language development, such as not responding to their own name or speaking only in single words, if at all • Repetitive and routine behaviors, such as walking in a specific pattern or insisting on eating the same meal every day • Difficulty making eye contact, such as focusing on a person's mouth when that person is speaking instead of their eyes, as is usual in most young children • Sensory problems, such as experiencing pain from certain sounds, like a ringing telephone or not reacting to intense cold or pain, certain sights, sounds, smells, textures, and tastes • Difficulty interpreting facial expressions, such as misreading or not noticing subtle facial cues, like a smile, wink, or grimace, that could help understand the nuances of social communication • Problems with expressing emotions, such as facial expressions, movements, tone of voice and gestures that are often vague or do not match what is said or felt • Fixation on parts of objects, such as focusing on a rotating wheel instead of playing with peers

(continued)

TABLE 6.11 Autism (*continued*)

	• Absence of pretend play, such as taking a long time to line up toys in a certain way, rather than playing with them • Difficulty interacting with peers, because they have a difficult time understanding that others have different information, feelings, and goals • Self-harm behavior, such as hitting head against a wall as a way of expressing disapproval • Sleep problems, such as falling asleep or staying asleep
Management/ treatment of autism	• Education and development including specialized classes and skilled training with therapists and other specialists • Applied behavioral analysis • Medications for symptoms • Changes in diet and supplements
Resources	National Alliance on Mental Illness (www.nami.org) Autism Speaks (www.autismspeaks.org) Autism Society of America (www.autism-society.org)

ASD, autism spectrum disorder.

TABLE 6.12 Dementia

Epidemiology	Dementia is a syndrome with multiple causes characterized by a decline in mental function, marked most commonly by memory impairment and a reduction in at least one other area of cognitive function such as reasoning, judgment, abstract thought, registration, comprehension, learning, task execution, and use of language.
	   Dementia is not a specific disease. It's an overall term that describes a wide range of symptoms associated with a decline in memory or other thinking skills severe enough to reduce a person's ability to perform everyday activities.
	   Dementia is caused by damage to brain cells. This damage interferes with the ability of brain cells to communicate with each other. When brain cells cannot communicate normally, thinking, behavior, and feelings can be affected.
	   When cells in a particular region are damaged, that region cannot carry out its functions normally.
	   In Alzheimer's disease, for example, high levels of certain proteins inside and outside brain cells make it hard for brain cells to stay healthy and to communicate with each *other*.

Types of dementia	The most common type of dementia is Alzheimer's disease; other types include vascular dementia, mixed dementia, dementia with Lewy bodies, and frontotemporal dementia.

(continued)

TABLE 6.12 Dementia (*continued*)

Risk factors	• Age • Genetics • Cardiovascular disease • Unhealthy eating habits Risk factors that may be reduced with proper management: • Depression • Medication side effects • Excess use of alcohol • Thyroid problems • Vitamin deficiencies
Diagnostic tests for dementia	There is no one test to diagnose dementia. Physicians conduct a physical exam, lab tests, and may conduct cognitive tests to evaluate memory, thinking, day-to-day function, and behavior to make a diagnosis of dementia. CT or MRI of the brain may be performed to rule out any other condition like stroke or tumors. Cognitive tests that may be used: • MMSE • Mini Cog • Mood assessment

Management of dementia	Treatment of dementia depends on its cause. In the case of most progressive dementias, including Alzheimer's disease, there is no cure and no treatment that slows or stops its progression.
	Medications
	• Cholinesterase inhibitors
	  ▪ Can address memory loss
	  ▪ Aricept
	  ▪ Used in early stages
	• Memantine
	  ▪ Can address memory loss
	  ▪ Namenda
	  ▪ Used for moderate to severe symptoms
	• Antipsychotics
	  ▪ May be prescribed for severe agitation and aggression
	  ▪ Efficacy is limited
	  ▪ Use puts the patient at risk of stroke and mortality
	Management should focus more on support care and services for the patient and caregiver. Clinical guidance advises non-pharmacologic interventions:
	• Early diagnosis
	• Management of other medical conditions
	• Education and counseling about the disease
	• Information about relevant supportive services
	• Observation of mood and behaviors
	  ▪ Environmental supports to mitigate aggression and agitation
	• End-of-life care

Resources	Alzheimer's Association (www.alz.org)

MMSE, Mini-Mental State Exam.

REFERENCES

American Psychological Association. (n.d.). Psychology topics. Retrieved from http://www.apa.org/topics/index.aspx

Godara, H., Hirbe, A., Nassif, M., Otepka, H. & Rosenstock, A. (Eds.). (2014). *The Washington manual of medical therapeutics* (34th ed.). Philadelphia, PA: Wolters Kluwer/Lippincott Williams & Wilkins.

National Alliance on Mental Illness. (n.d.). Mental health conditions. Retrieved from https://www.nami.org/Learn-More/Mental-Health-Conditions

Stein, D. J., Phillips, K. A., Bolton, D., & Fulford, K. W. M. (2010). What is a mental/psychiatric disorder? From *DSM-IV* to *DSM-V*. *Psychological Medicine*, *40*, 1759–1765. doi:10.1017/S0033291709992261

PART III

Strategies for Optimal Patient Communication and Outcomes With Integrated Case Management

Addressing Social Determinants: Clinical Versus Nonclinical Issues

Rebecca Perez
Kathleen Fraser

Our lives begin to end the day we become silent about things that matter.

—Martin Luther King, Jr.

OBJECTIVES

- Describe the interaction of clinical and nonclinical issues impacting patient engagement and adherence
- Recognize the role of social issues in care and transition plan adherence
- Identify social determinants through the integrated case management process
- Understand the impact of nonclinical and social issues as contributors to hospital admission

The Centers for Medicare and Medicaid (CMS) and National Quality Forum's (NQF's) Triple Aim recognize that social factors have a direct impact on an individual's ability to be healthy. Individuals with a low socioeconomic status are generally less healthy than those with a higher socioeconomic status. Addressing social determinants of health (SDOH) must be addressed as a priority if we want to impact the overall health of the patients we serve.

What Are Social Determinants of Health?

How we take care of ourselves and how we stay healthy is well known by most:

- Go to school

- Consume a healthy diet: low fat, high amounts of fruit and vegetables, low sugar intake

- Exercise regularly

- Do not smoke or use any form of tobacco

- Get recommended immunizations

- Get 6 to 8 hours of sleep every night

- See a primary care physician for well and sick visits

These steps will keep us physically healthy but we also need to have social and environmental supports to maintain health. We may not correlate that health starts in the places where we live, work, and go to school (U.S. Department of Health and Human Services [DHHS], 2017). Where and how we access the resources needed to be healthy should be located in our homes, communities, in the quality of our schools, in a safe workplace, in access to clean air, water, and food; and in good social interactions and relationships (2017). Some Americans are healthier than others, and that, in part, is due to conditions in which we live.

To promote good health for all Americans, we need to create social and physical environments that support good health. The interferences keeping Americans from being healthy can be directly related to SDOH. SDOH are defined as conditions that affect a wide range of health, function, quality of life, and health risk (2017). The environment in which a person is born, lives, works, plays, worships, and ages as well as social, economic, and physical conditions all impact the ability to be healthy (2017).

Stability of "place" refers to the physical attributes of where a person lives. Patterns of social engagement and a sense of well-being and security influence "place" (2017). Having resources to promote stability of place, social support, safety, and well-being are what impact health outcomes.

According to DHHS, examples of SDOH include the following:

- Availability of resources to meet daily needs
  - Safe housing
  - Access to food
- Availability of, and access to, educational, economic, and job opportunities
- Access to health care services
- Quality of education and job training
- Availability of community-based resources in support of community living and access to leisure activities
- Transportation options
- Public safety
- Social supports
- Presence of discrimination, racism, distrust of government
- Exposure to crime, violence, lack of community commitment/cooperation
- Concentrated poverty and related stresses
- Residential segregation
- Language/literacy
- Access to technology
  - Cell phones
  - Internet
- Cultural practices

Physical determinants include:

- Environmental: lack of greenspace (trees, grass), climate change
- Built environment: buildings, sidewalks, bike lanes, and roads
- Workplace, schools, and recreational settings
- Housing and community design

- Exposure to toxic substances and other physical hazards
- Physical barriers, especially for those with disabilities
- Aesthetic impact: lighting, trees, public benches

Many of these determinants are outside the scope of a case manager's control or ability to intervene, but it is important to understand the impact. The determinants that can be impacted will be listed here and are crucial components that directly impact the health of an individual and can be impacted by specific case management interventions (2017).

FIGURE 7.1 Social determinants of health.

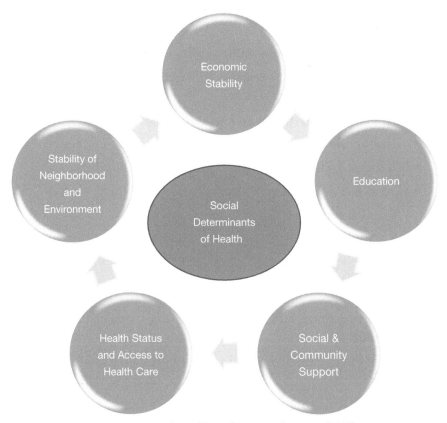

Source: From U.S. Department of Health and Human Services (2017).

Economic Stability

Through a network of available community resources, case managers can help patients connect with resources to assist with the acquisition of food, for example, application for food stamps or access to food pantries, payment of utilities, and affordable housing. For those individuals seeking employment assistance, we can connect the patient to vocational resources. Reducing the stress of financial concerns allows the patient to better focus on health issues. We should work with our team members and the community to develop a list of resources that can easily and quickly be referenced so that prompt assistance can be provided.

Education

Again, having resources available related to education can assist a patient in reaching a personal goal of advancing education. An individual's ability to advance his or her education may open the door for improving status in life by providing employment opportunities not previously available. This may mean achieving a general education diploma (GED), entrance to community college, university, or trade school. Personal educational advancement may lead to improved financial stability and improved quality of life.

Social and Community Support

Patients with complex health needs require social supports to better manage health needs. Without social support, their health and ability to self-manage are at risk. For patients with family or other available social supports, we need to encourage the involvement and participation of these supports. Patients may refuse this involvement and we ultimately must respect a patient's decision, but we can certainly continue to encourage social support involvement, especially if the patient struggles to manage his or her conditions. We would use our motivational interviewing skills to help the patient begin to think about the benefits of additional support.

When a patient has no visible means of support, no family or reliable friends, we can make recommendations to participate in support groups, join community social groups, or faith-based communities. These can be very effective at supplementing the absence of related social supports.

Health Status and Access to Health Care

As case managers, assisting our patients to get health care and services to improve their health is a priority. However, we must recognize the barriers that may be preventing stable health and mitigate the interference and risks related to poor health. The inability to access needed health care and services can be related, for example, to limited access to providers due to geographic reasons or language barriers; limited insurance benefits like high deductibles; lack of mental health coverage; lack of transportation to get to appointments; providers with limited appointment schedules or office hours; and of most concern, a patient's distrust of health care providers.

We must diligently work to remove these barriers. Our place of practice: health plan, insurance company, hospital, long-term care, independent practice, may limit us in what benefits and services are reimbursable or covered for the patient. Some managed Medicaid and Medicare plans see the value in providing services like non-emergent transportation to provider appointments. However, if non-emergent transportation is not a covered benefit for your patient, you will need to explore other resources that could assist your patient in keeping medical appointments. Another strategy could be assisting the patient to get an appointment time that would be more convenient for available transportation. Patients whose primary language is not English may need help in finding a physician who speaks their primary language, or finding a medical translator to interpret provider visits. Patients who live in rural areas have an especially difficult time finding providers, especially specialty and behavioral health providers. We must provide the assistance to find providers and schedule appointments. When multiple appointments are needed, for example, appointment to see a physician and completion of diagnostic tests, or, a medical appointment and counseling appointment, every effort should be made to get these appointments scheduled to be completed on the same day so that the patient is not making multiple long trips to complete appointments.

During the assessment process, we determine the patient's understanding of his or her conditions and prescribed treatment plan. The patient's level of health literacy directly impacts this understanding. We must ascertain what the patient knows and understands, what the physician has imparted, and then bring this all together to help the patient understand, using language that is easily comprehended. This means using nonmedical and simple terms, analogies, and perhaps even visuals.

Stability of Neighborhood and Environment

Case managers do not typically "build" healthy environments but can certainly support what a community may offer. Access to healthy foods may mean guiding your patient to shopping at a local farmer's market that accepts food stamps to purchase fresh, locally grown and typically affordable fruits and vegetables. If the patient is residing in housing that is in disrepair, infested with insects or vermin, is in a high crime area, or is a victim of abuse or neglect, we have a responsibility to help the patient find safe housing. A safe environment reduces the risk of poor health, injury, and trauma.

Assessing the presence of social determinants and risk occurs as part of the integrated, comprehensive assessment. Social concerns are included in the four domains assessed when using an integrated approach. We may find that a patient's health conditions are stable at present but may be at risk due to the presence of social determinants. Addressing the social concerns as a priority can result in continued health stabilization and prevention of complications.

The social concerns assessment for integrated case management using the ICM-CAG tool reviews the history (past 6 months) of a patient's ability to work or go to school. Source of income not from a job would also be included. Working includes being a stay-at-home partner who manages a household and/or children. Social relationships encompass the quality and the presence of active engagement with family, friends and coworkers. Status (past 30 days) examines the patient's support system: family, friends, or others who are available to assist the patient when needed, and the environment in which they live safely. The safety of the environment includes the ability to pay for a mortgage, rent, utilities, food, medications, clothing, and so forth. The patient's history and status are evaluated to determine if the patient is at risk of social deterioration in the next 3 to 6 months if case management interventions do not continue.

Let us look at case studies related to SDOH.

CASE STUDY 1

Cassie is a 6-year-old girl living in subsidized housing with her grandmother and brother Sam. The apartment building was built in the early 1960s, is in disrepair, and cockroach infestations are frequent. Mold is visible in the building hallways due to leaking pipes in the ceiling. Cassie has asthma, is in the emergency department (ED) at least once per month with exacerbations, and often misses school.

What interventions are appropriate to reduce Cassie's visits to the ED? ■ ■ ■

CASE STUDY 2

Brittany is a 32-year-old woman who is in the ED three to four times per month on average with complaints of abdominal pain. Brittany currently lives with her boyfriend who has a violent temper and physically assaults her. The hospital ED has referred Brittany to a social worker but Brittany has never contacted the social worker.

What interventions might be appropriate for Brittany to reduce her risk of injury? ■ ■ ■

CASE STUDY 3

George is a 72-year-old gentleman living alone since his wife Sarah passed away 2 years ago. George has diabetes but the co-pay for his medications and testing supplies forces him to choose between getting his medications and supplies or paying for utilities and groceries. George will buy his testing supplies every other month and buy only canned soup at the grocery store to be able to meet all his expenses.

What interventions would help George to meet all his financial obligations but also access his medicines and testing supplies? ■ ■ ■

Our current system lacks the infrastructure and reimbursement processes to implement programs that address social determinants (

FIGURE 7.2 U.S. health care spending on direct medical services.

"By some estimates, more than 95% of the trillion dollars spent on health care in the United States each year funds direct medical services, even though 60% of preventable deaths are rooted in modifiable behaviors and exposures that occur in the community."

Source: From Alley et al. (2016).

(Alley, Asomuhga, Conway, & Sangahavi, 2016). Health systems are being held accountable to improve outcomes and reduce the cost of care, but the tools and interventions needed to address community and social factors are unavailable (Figure 7.2).

Development of a systematic approach to address social determinants will reduce health care costs, especially for those most at risk. The CMS recently announced a 5-year, $157 million program called Accountable Health Communities to be implemented in 2018 (Alley et al., 2016). Comprehensive screenings will be conducted to assess for health-related social needs like homelessness, poor housing quality, inability to pay rent or mortgage, food insecurity, difficulty paying for utilities, evidence of intimate partner violence, elder abuse, child neglect and maltreatment, and lack of transportation (Alley et al., 2016).

The ability for any community to meet these needs will widely vary. As a result, the Accountable Health Communities demonstration project has been designed to track the readiness of communities through Awareness, Assistance, and Alignment (Alley et al., 2016). The program participants are termed "bridge organizations" and can be community organizations, clinical networks, or other organizations that demonstrate a strong relationship with both clinical and community partners (Alley et al., 2016). The project's goal should include validation of increased awareness of community services, and reduction in costs related to ED visits and admissions. Providing navigation assistance to beneficiaries in accessing services will reduce the overall cost of care: ED and admissions, supported by a combination of community service navigation and community partner alignment (Alley et al., 2016).

The Accountable Health Communities model is a method by which the CMS hopes to demonstrate a growing emphasis on population health and whether savings will materialize through the collaboration of health care providers and their respective communities. For us as case managers, being aware of this initiative is important so that we can perhaps gain new insight into better methods of intervention to improve the social challenges faced by our patients. We will be watching for the results of this demonstration project in the next 5 years.

REFERENCES

Alley, D. E., Asomuhga, C. N., Conway, P. H., & Sangahavi, D. M. (2016). Accountable health communities: Addressing social needs through Medicare and Medicaid. *The New England Journal of Medicine, 374,* 8–11. doi:10.1056/NEJMp1512532

U.S. Department of Health and Human Services. (2017). *Healthy People 2020.* Retrieved from https://www.healthypeople.gov/2020/topics-objectives/topic/social-determinants-of-health

Motivational Interviewing and Shared Decision Making for the Medically Complex Patient and Family Caregiver

Jos Dobber
Corine Latour

Therapeutic engagement is a prerequisite for everything that follows.

—Miller and Rollnick (2013)

OBJECTIVES

- Able to define the principles of motivational interviewing and coaching
- Understand the intervention and tasks associated with the integrated case management process
- Relate patient engagement and adherence to motivational coaching
- Understand patient-centered preference engagement and share decision-making activities

Complex patients do not always seem to make good health decisions, especially not from the professional's point of view. Health behaviors such as treatment adherence and healthy food habits can help to improve these patients' conditions and their quality of life, if they would make good choices. Although one would expect a person to stop smoking after having a heart attack, the truth is that about 30% to 50% of the patients continue to smoke (Chow et al., 2010; Jorstad et al., 2013). The case manager is in the position to support the patients in making sensible health behavior decisions. For this, motivational interviewing (MI) provides an attitude and skills. The case manager guides the patient, based on a trusting relationship between the patient and the case manager, in which the patient's perspective on his or her health problems and health behaviors is the starting point for the case manager. The patient and the case manager work together in such a way that the patient is actively involved in his or her own care and in the decision making regarding health problems and treatment plans (Berger & Villaume, 2013). Hereto a combination of MI and shared decision making (SDM) enables the case manager to fulfill this role.

Principles of Motivation and MI

Often, professionals such as case managers assess the need for behavioral change in patients. Some patients may recognize this need and are ready to change, while others may feel ambivalent about change or resist change. The first group is considered to be motivated for change, whereas the second and third groups may frequently be regarded as lacking motivation. Remarkably, all three groups may profit from a skilled MI approach by their case manager.

In MI theory (Miller & Rollnick, 2002), motivation comprises three critical components: willingness to change/importance of the change; ability to change/confidence in the change; readiness to change. Each component is a building block for intrinsic motivation. Since the patient is an autonomous person, and the behavioral change is supposed to be a sustainable change, MI aims to stimulate intrinsic motivation: behavioral change for the patient's own good reasons.

"Motivational interviewing is a person-centered counseling style for addressing the common problem of ambivalence about change" (Miller & Rollnick, 2013, p. 29). It is an effective intervention to enhance motivation for behavioral change (Lundahl et al., 2013). When case managers use MI, they influence the patient's willingness, ability, and readiness to elicit intrinsic motivation and to enable behavioral change. For this, the case manager uses MI techniques and communicates in an empathic style. The language of change plays a major role in MI. Based on Bem's theory of self-perception (1967), MI aims to evoke intrinsic patient motivation by eliciting patient verbal expressions in favor of change. These patient expressions are called "change talk" (in favor of change), which contrasts with "sustain talk" (in favor of status quo).

If the patient is already willing to make the behavioral change, the case manager can move on to the change plan, and support the patient to concretize the plan in actions and with a time frame. They may also identify potential helpful sources. Exploring possible barriers for changing, and discussing ways to avoid or handle these barriers (coping planning), may also be an important issue. Finally, if the patient has already made some steps to change his or her behavior, the case manager can strengthen the motivation of the patient by affirming these efforts, and reflecting the patient's increasing self-control over his or her health behavior.

Patients who do not think their (potential) health problem is important will not see the need to change, so the first step for the case manager is to enhance the perceived importance. Sometimes patients are regarded as "not motivated," while this may be a matter of finding the goal or value for which the patient is motivated. "Exercise" may not attract the patient, while he or she sure wants to be able again to climb the stairs in his or her own house, and sleeping in his or her bedroom.

In contrast to patients who are ready to change, or those who resist change, ambivalent patients express conflicting motivations on behavioral change: "I like my burgers, not so good for my health I know, I should lose some pounds, but that's how I am." Most health care professionals are inclined to take up the healthy part: "Yes, like you said, you should change your food habits." The ambivalent person, however, sees two sides. And since the health care professional is telling him or her to change his or her diet, the person feels forced to plead for the other side, which was ignored by the professional: "Well I'm not like that; with us, everyone eats burgers." So, the professional reached the opposite effect of what was intended the patient argues against change (Berger & Bertram, 2015; Miller & Rollnick, 2013). The MI reaction would have been to reflect both sides of the ambivalence: "It's difficult to imagine yourself not eating burgers, though you know it would benefit your health to cut down on fast food and lose some weight."

MI Spirit

MI may verge on some sort of mental shift from the case manager. The case manager should take a step back and try to understand the way the patient sees his or her health problems and the ways of dealing with them (Berger & Villaume, 2013). This is the spirit of MI: acceptance, collaboration, compassion, and evocation (Miller & Rollnick, 2013). Through this spirit, the case manager communicates the partnership with the patient. That relation is not defined as "an active expert helping a passive patient," but rather as "two experts working together as equals." After all, the patient is the expert in his or her own life and knows best what works for him or her and what does not.

Change Talk and Sustain Talk

Through change talk (in favor of change) and sustain talk (in favor of status quo), the patient expresses his or her reasons, doubts, cognitions, and health beliefs related to health behavior. In MI, there are seven types of change talk and sustain talk: desire, reasons, need, ability, commitment, activation, and taking steps (see Table 8.1). "I know, I must quit smoking" is a need-pro change statement, while "I can't stop smoking, not in my house where my wife and sons smoke their cigarettes" is a statement with two types of sustain talk: inability to change and a reason to resist change. Since change talk functions as the main working mechanism of MI, case managers should evoke patient change talk, and try to avoid patient sustain talk without ignoring it.

A part of the sustain talk derives from the explanatory model of the patient for his or her health problems. Another part of the sustain talk originates from the patient's reaction (e.g., fear) to his or her health problems. This means that the case manager, to be able to influence the patient's motivation, needs to understand the patient's view on his or her health and health problems (cf. Berger & Villaume, 2013).

Change talk and sustain talk also function as a signal for the case manager on the progress of the patient's process in becoming more motivated. It is important to listen to the patient and tune the pace and the course of the conversation to the patient's motivational process. If the patient expresses unsolicited change talk, then mostly there is no need to make a decision balance listing the pros and cons of the current

TABLE 8.1 Change Talk and Sustain Talk

	EXAMPLE CHANGE TALK	EXAMPLE SUSTAIN TALK
DARN: preparatory change talk		
Desire statement	"I don't want to live on junk food anymore."	"I want to eat like I've done my whole life."
Ability statement	"I can cook healthy food."	"I can hardly boil an egg."
Reason statement	"I have to lose weight."	"I like my food butter-baked."
Need statement	"I need to eat much healthier than I do now."	"I don't need to eat vegetables on a daily basis."
CAT: mobilizing change talk		
Commitment	"Starting today, I'll cook the food myself instead of taking microwave-food."	"Drop the subject, I am stopping the healthy food diet."
Activation	"I'm willing to cook healthy meals on a regular basis."	"I'm not ready to change my way of cooking."
Taking steps	"I bought the healthy food cookbook."	"I didn't go to the appointment with the dietician."

health behavior or of the behavioral change. After all, there is change talk already to continue the conversation in a productive direction, while composing a decision balance means evoking both change talk and sustain talk.

Patient utterances of change talk and sustain talk can refer to the (non)importance of behavioral change and to the (lack of) confidence in the change. Patients can be willing to change, but may have no idea how to accomplish this. In complex patients, sometimes other (physical, mental, situational) conditions have to change first to make the behavioral change possible. Some patients are able to take small steps with a (small) personalized goal for each step. However, for patients who are willing to change, but without confidence in their ability, no change will occur, and eventually the willingness will also disappear: "Why should I want to change if I can't?"

Ambivalence

Ambivalence is a special pattern in which the patient expresses motivations both pro and contra change. However, ambivalence is a normal phenomenon and does not mean that the patient is not motivated. If the patient expresses ambivalence, the case manager should reflect this ambivalence, reflecting both the pro and the contra side of the ambivalence expressed by the patient. This should be done in an accepting and nonjudgmental way: "So you are kind of on two tracks at the same time. Smoking helps you dealing with stress, but on the other hand you want to stop smoking because that is better for your health." Depending on the patient's reaction to the case manager's reflection, the case manager and patient can explore the ambivalence to support the patient in solving it. By contrast, a persuasive reaction telling the patient that continuing smoking will indeed cause health problems would probably trigger the patient to argue in favor of the other side of the ambivalence (Miller & Rollnick, 2013): "I can't, too much stress."

MI: Four Processes

MI is goal oriented; it aims for behavioral change. While performing MI, the case manager tunes the patient's process of becoming (more) motivated and the case manager's process of promoting intrinsic motivation, through four MI processes: engaging, focusing, evoking, and planning (Miller & Rollnick, 2013). These central processes help the case manager navigate effectively through MI conversations about behavioral change.

Engaging

Relation building is the starting point of MI. Every person wants to be treated with respect, and wants to be taken seriously. If the patient perceives that the case manager understands his or her problems and perspectives, is listened to and treated with respect and concern, this helps him or her to explore the situation and reasons and motives for his or her current health behavior. A trusting relationship is fostered by the case manager's skills, such as reflective listening, asking open-ended questions, showing empathy, acceptance, and understanding. By

TABLE 8.2 The Four Main Conversational Techniques — OARS

Open-ended questions	Determines the topic, and invites the patient to elaborate
Affirming	Acknowledges what is already good, supports, and encourages
Reflecting	Simple reflections: rephrasing what the patient just said
	Complex reflections: giving the essence of the meaning the patient meant to communicate, and sometimes going one step further by including what the patient did not say, but what can be the next step in the thought process
Summarizing	Complex reflection that connects previous patient statements on the target behavior

contrast, this relationship may be hindered by focusing on actual facts in the patient's story (ignoring the patient's perception), the appearance of a question–answer pattern, and by taking up the expert role. The four main conversational techniques to build rapport are displayed in Table 8.2.

Focusing

Determining the health behavioral change goal is an important process. Though the establishment of such a goal seems obvious, frequently the patient's change goals do not coincide with the case manager's change goals for the patient. So, the focusing process is about finding the patient's change goals and finding ground to work together on a common purpose (cf. Miller & Rollnick, 2013; e.g., "being able to button up my shirt" or "tying my shoelaces" instead of "losing weight").[1] Focusing also means that the case manager ensures that the health behavioral change goal stays at the center of the conversation.

Evoking

The essence of the evoking process is eliciting and exploring the patient's own good motives for change. This is an important working mechanism of MI; if patients hear themselves argue for change, they convince themselves to change (Miller & Rollnick, 2013), and their own argumentation may also change their self-perception ("I'm a mother, should not be a drinker, I can work through this"; Bem, 1967; Miller & Rollnick, 2002). The four main conversational techniques (Table 8.2) are powerful techniques in evoking the patient's intrinsic motivation.

It is important to notice that the evoking process is not meant as a way to manipulate the patient. In MI, the case manager guides the patient to find his or her own reasons, motives, values, goals for change, and not those of the case manager.

Planning

The planning process is about helping patients to move on to actual change when the patient is willing and ready to change. Not all patients want or need help with planning, and pushing them may do more harm than good to their motivation. But often a small concrete plan supports the patient to envision the change. As with evoking, the plan should be the patient's plan, not the case manager's. The case manager's task is to support the patient making his or her own plan, asking questions such as: "What would be your first step?"; "Who could help you?"; "What are barriers you might encounter?"; and providing information at the request of the patient.

Conversations on motivation are not linear, and, although there is a logical order, these processes do not appear purely sequentially. It is important to engage first, but while focusing, engaging still remains important. And, while planning, focus on the change goal remains important. Miller and Rollnick (2013) use the metaphor of stair steps: each process rests on the fundament of previous processes, and previous processes are still active supporting the following processes. Also, during the conversation, the patient and the case manager sometimes move up and down the stair steps, depending on both the course of the conversation and the development of the trusting relationship between them.

Consistent Practice

For case managers, MI may be a reference method, a patient-centered way of care giving; hence, the effectiveness of this care depends on the MI consistency of the execution. In the following section, there is a short description of the MI posture and MI core skills (see also Allison, Bes, & Rose, 2012).

The Core Values of MI

Miller and Rollnick (2013) emphasize the importance of the core values of MI: the MI spirit, a composition of partnership, acceptance, evocation, and compassion. They describe MI spirit as the mind-set and heart-set of the practitioner. The case manager is not someone who can change the behavior of the patient, and does not have an answer to all the problems and concerns of the patient. However, the health behavioral change can be facilitated through a partnership between the case manager and the patient, in which both persons respect each other, and in which the starting point is (understanding) the patient's perspective of his or her health problems and the reaction to that.

A second characteristic of the MI spirit is the acceptance of the unique person the patient is. This does not mean that the case manager agrees with all the patient's actions, but the case manager tries to understand the person from the patient's perspective and does not judge the person. Respecting the patient as an autonomous person is also part of acceptance; hence "making patients do things" is an important "don't" in MI. By contrast, affirmation for the strengths of the patient and for his or her efforts and attempts shows the case manager's acceptance of the patient.

Evocation is the third characteristic of MI spirit that emphasizes the resources of the patient: the person already has much of what he or she needs, and is not "missing something" that the case manager can give. Compassion is the fourth characteristic of MI spirit. The case manager feels involved with the patient, is caring, acknowledges that the patient is more than his or her health problems, and is committed to the best interest of the patient.

The characteristics of the MI spirit lead to a collaboration between the patient and the case manager, in which the patient feels free to express ideas, concerns, and goals. Together, the patient and the case manager focus on the goals upon which they have both agreed.

Empathy and Collaboration

Accurate empathy, showing the case manager's effort to understand the patient's perspective and his or her personal meanings, is not only a core value of MI but also a skill. Through empathic reflections, the case manager creates a working atmosphere in which the patient feels safe to express concerns and to ask the questions he or she did not ask other health professionals. The empathy cultivates rapport with the patient, but, when persevered though the conversation, averts discord. At the same time, empathy contributes to the effectiveness of the information the case manager provides to the patient. Patients are more likely to believe the information given by people they like.

During the conversation, both partners should sense the partnership: working together as equals on a mutually agreed goal (cf. Allison et al., 2012). The agenda, ideas, and concerns of the patient are taken seriously, and are addressed in the conversation. All health decisions are reached through the principles of SDM.

Focus on the Behavioral Change

MI is a purposeful conversation. The case manager intentionally directs the conversation to the behavioral change. Depending on the individual patient and the progress of the conversation, the case manager selects conversational techniques and strategies that are most appropriate. While active listening may fit best at the start of the conversation, the case manager should be able to switch to reflect the patient's ambivalence and explore this ambivalence instantly if applicable. Discussing the importance of specific health behavior for the patient, or discussing options, giving information and advice, planning, all these techniques can be applied if it seems the most appropriate at that particular moment in the conversation. So, case managers need to have the flexibility to employ the activity that contributes best to the patient's motivational process, and that equips the patient to make his or her own well-informed decisions.

Self-Control

The patient's experience of control serves several functions in an MI conversation. First, it is important that the patient sees him- or herself as the person who makes the decisions on health behaviors. The case manager encourages the patient to take responsibility for both the health behavior and the decision making.

Second, patients usually do not like the idea that other people, like health professionals, are making the decisions and telling them to "quit smoking, do more exercise, take medications as prescribed." So, if patients sense that health decisions are made for them by the case manager, they may react defensively ("Nothing wrong with my food habits") or disengage from the conversation. If signals like this appear, the case manager should take a step back and reconsider his or her strategy. The acknowledgment of the patient's autonomy through emphasizing the patient's control over the decision making helps to get back on track.

Third, sometimes the patient has already taken some steps to change health behavior, and seems to have found a way in which this new health behavior fits in his or her daily routines. In this situation, the case manager affirms the patient for taking these steps, and reflects that this shows how the patient is taking control over his or her health behavior (Patient: "I've stopped having ice cream all the time. Now I allow myself only one ice cream a week, and tell you what: now I'm really tasting this ice cream, I enjoy it so much! But I also enjoy the other days, seeing that I'm strong enough, taking some fruit or just water instead." Case manager: "Good for you! You've really accomplished something important! Now you find yourself in control, you are managing your food habits in a way that really fits you."). By this affirmation and reflection, the case manager fosters the patient's cognition of self-control.

Evocation

The case manager employs MI to evoke the patient's own motivation for health behavioral change. If ambivalence blocks the behavioral change, the case manager guides the patient to move ahead and, by listening to his or her own argumentation, resolves the ambivalence. The argumentation of the patient comprises six kinds of statements: Desire, Ability, Reasons, Need, Commitment, Activation, Taking Steps (DARN-CAT). The first four types of statements are seen as preparatory change talk. If the patient says "I know I should take these pills everyday," this does not mean that he or she will take the medication daily. The statement only expresses some kind of importance, but, since it is the patient who recognizes this importance, the need statement is a building block in the patient's own argumentation to eventually make a decision on taking or not taking the medication as prescribed. The other three types of statements are mobilizing change talk (Miller & Rollnick, 2013).

Ambivalent patients see two sides of the behavioral change, and in the conversation they will utter both change talk and sustain talk. The case manager reflects both, but gives more attention to the change talk. (Patient: "There's lots of reasons why I should exercise, but I'm just too lazy for it." Case manager: "You're too lazy. And you mentioned something about reasons for exercise, tell me more about it: what would be the best reason?") Evocative questions and complex reflections are the most important tools in evocation. When the patient has told the best reason to exercise, the case manager reflects the reason, and may ask another question to elaborate on the best reason. (Patient: "I have no condition, when we're going somewhere I always lag behind." Case manager: "Your friends' conditions are way better; where does this leave you?" Patient: "Well sometimes I just stay home instead of going out with them.") The case manager is not convincing the patient, but just reflecting and asking questions. As a consequence, the patient is arguing against a status quo. Forming good reflections is a powerful technique. Good reflections do not exactly reflect the patient's statement, but go one step further: what did the patient mean that he or she has not said? Or: What would be the next step in the patient's thought process? So, reflections have the power to help patients move forward in their thought processes, because the patient's thought process is the starting point of the reflection. Also, a skillfully worded reflection sounds like a thought unit of the patient, while the starting point and the formulation of a question reflect the thought process of the question-asking case manager. Apodaca et al. (2016) found that reflections and open-ended questions elicit both change talk and sustain talk, probably mainly while exploring the patient's ambivalence.

Beside these techniques, the case manager also has the option to employ specific strategies that usually open a door to change talk. A description of these strategies can be found in the paragraph: "Optional MI components."

Recognizing the urge or importance of the health behavior is key to willing to change. However, not all patients sense the importance of the behavior, so they do not perceive the need for behavioral change. If this is the case, in MI the case manager tries to create discrepancy. The case manager explores whether the health behavior can be linked to an important value or goal of the patient. In many cases, by carefully listening to the patient in previous conversations or earlier in the current conversation, the case manager may already know what the goals and the values of the patient are.

An example is a 67-year-old woman, living alone, small social network, feeling lonely, overweight (BMI = 34), and having a serious heart condition after a myocardial infarction a few months ago. She tells the case manager that she changed her food habits and is on a healthy diet now, but she does not really lose weight. The case manager asks her about her shopping this morning, and she tells that she bought vegetables, meat, some fruit, and some candy.

Case manager: "Why candy?"

Patient: "I can't resist buying it; it's delicious you know."

Case manager: "It's hard not to buy candy when you think of its taste. How about fruit?"

Patient: "I've tried that, but lately I bought grapes and ate them all within the hour. And besides, I need to have candy for my grandchildren. But if I have candy, I can't resist taking some myself."

Case manager: "They expect to get some when they visit you. Do they come every day?"

Patient: "Yes, all four of them live real close. And after school they always drop by and find their way to the candy. I can't think of disappointing them."

Case manager: So, on one hand it frustrates you to buy candy and on the other hand you're afraid to fail your grandchildren."

Patient: "Yes, it is like that . . . I don't know, what can I do?"

Case manager: "The kids are your daughter's?"

Patient: "Two daughters. They both have two kids."

Case manager: "And where do they stand? Your daughters I mean?"

Patient: "They hate it. My youngest daughter especially, I know her lines by heart: Too much candy for the kids . . . No need for candy everyday . . . Mum, they are my kids, when are you going to listen to me . . ."

Case manager: "What do you make of that?"

Patient: "Nothing, it's just something she keeps saying."

Case manager: "She keeps saying it. How does it affect your relation with her?"

Patient: "Well, it is not very social if that is what you mean."

Case manager: "It is not as good as it was before."

Patient: "No, we did have quite an intimate relationship as a matter of fact."

Case manager: "And you would like that back."

Patient: "You mean . . . would it help . . . the candy . . .? And what do I say to my grandchildren?"

The case manager relates the candy to the patient's relationship with her daughter. Next, the patient and the case manager can explore whether that relationship is important enough to change for. It is the patient who must come to a conclusion about this, not the case manager.

Optional MI Components

Sometimes an optional MI component helps learning about the patient's perspective, the occurrence of the target behavior in daily life, or to evoke change talk. These components are strategies that may be helpful in a conversation. The use of the components depends on the course of the conversation, and on the fit of the component with the case manager's style. See Table 8.3 for a summarized overview of these components.

A Typical Day/Typical Week

This strategy can be used to replace the question–answer structure of an anamnesis, or to gain insight in the presence of the target behavior in the day-to-day life of the patient.

Ask the patient to walk you through a normal day (or normal week). It is best to ask for a concrete and recent day (yesterday), that the patient still remembers well. Take 2 to 10 minutes for this component. Start by saying "You got up at . . .? And then?" The patient will take off by this prompt and tell about yesterday. Ask questions if the patient's story needs clarification ("Did you climb the stairs, or did you go by elevator?"), but don't interrupt too much: the patient is walking you through the day, it is not an examination. Stay interested, increase or decrease the pace of the patient's story if necessary (Rollnick, Miller, & Butler, 2007).

TABLE 8.3 Overview of the Optional Components

Typical day/typical week	Provides insight in the presence of the target behavior in the patient's daily life
Balance sheet	Evokes both change talk and sustain talk, but may help to explore the ambivalence, especially when there are hardly any change talk statements
Importance ruler/confidence ruler	Evokes statements about importance/willingness, or about confidence/ability
Querying extremes	Evokes change talk if the patient doesn't seem to want to change in the present
Exploring goals and values	Helps finding out what may be worthwhile to change for
Looking back/looking forward	Stimulates the envision of the benefits of the change
Giving information and advice	If properly done, it may help to influence the patient's sense making
Change plan	Increases the chance of a successful change

Balance Sheet

If the change talk does not come, then the case manager may consider the use of a balance sheet. This component should not be carried out routinely, because it not only evokes change talk, but also sustain talk.

Draw a line on a sheet of paper to divide it into halves, one side for the "pros of the current health behavior," the other side for the "cons of the current health behavior." Start by the pros; this evokes sustain talk of the patient. Reflect the pros mentioned by the patient, but do not elaborate (too much) on the pros. Write each pro down in two or three words; continue by asking: "What else?" After completing the pros, shift to the cons, which evoke change talk. The cons may contain motives for behavioral change, if the patient perceives the motive as important enough to change for. The consequence of this is that the case manager takes the time to explore the importance of each con mentioned. For this purpose, the case manager reflects the con, and adds a follow-up question: "Not taking your pills may affect your health condition. What could happen to your health?" Guided by the patient's reaction, the case manager decides whether to continue on this subject or to move on to the next con. If the subject seems important, the case manager uses open questions and complex reflections to evoke change talk. After finishing the cons-side of the decision balance, the case manager summarizes both sides: "On one hand, you don't want to take your medication because. . . ., but on the other hand, not using medication may affect your health, and sometimes you find yourself wondering. . . ."

It is also possible to draw four boxes: (1) pros of current health behavior; (2) cons of current health behavior; (3) cons of health behavioral change; (4) pros of health behavioral change. However, patients may regard box 1 as (almost) the same as box 3, and box 2 (almost) completely overlapping with box 4. An example is the patient who states that in box 1, drinking alcohol makes him feel at ease, and mentions in box 3 that if he could not take his beer, that would make him tense, because he needs alcohol to feel at ease.

Importance Ruler

The importance ruler is a simple evocative question. The procedure is the case manager asking "On a scale from 0 to 10, where 0 means not important at all, and 10 means most important, how important is this change for you?" The patient will answer with a number between 0 and 10, say 5. The case manager reflects this in a neutral tone: "Five." The value of this strategy is in the follow-up question: "Five. Why are you not at four?" By mentioning one number lower, the patient will explain that the behavioral change is more important than a 4. So, the patient explains the reasons and need to change, which means: change talk. If the follow-up question would be "Why are you not at six?" this would evoke arguments why the change is not so important: sustain talk.

Confidence Ruler

The confidence ruler is the same kind of evocative question as the importance ruler, but focuses on self-efficacy. Obviously, the question would be: "If you would make this change, how would you score your confidence to make a successful change? On a scale from 0 to 10, where 0 means not confident at all, and 10 means very confident, how would you score?"

Querying Extremes

By asking, "How would this change make your life better?" or, "What would be the worst things that could happen if you continue to go on as you do now?" the case manager may evoke change talk, especially if the patient does not seem to want to change at the present.

Exploring Goals and Values

Goals and values can be powerful triggers for behavioral change. Goals and values tell the case manager what it is that most motivates the patient. Although sometimes it might seem obvious to the case manager how the present health behavior may interfere with goals and values of the patient, this relation often is not so clear for patients. In MI, it is important that the patient him- or herself draws the conclusion that changing health behavior helps reaching his or her goals or values.

Imagine a well-educated patient with chronic vulnerability for psychosis. She has a description for antipsychotic medication, but she values her autonomy and wants "to beat psychosis in her own strength." So, if she feels fine, she discontinues her medication, and after a while she suffers from another psychosis. The case manager knows that "keeping a job" is also an important goal for this patient. The frequent relapses, however, make it impossible to stay in a job, and the patient finds this very frustrating. The case manager applies the decisional balance component on long-term medication adherence, and the patient knows a lot of cons (not natural, side effects, want to be stronger than psychosis). On the pro-side the patient mentions only "longer periods free of psychosis." The follow-up question of the case manager is: "What means being free of psychosis for you?" Patient: "Staying out of hospitals, living a normal life." The case manager invites the patient to elaborate on that: "What do you do in normal life what you can't do when you're suffering from psychosis?" This question triggers the reasoning of the patient, and quickly she arrives at the conclusion: "So, taking my medication helps me to keep my job."

Looking Forward/Looking Back

A simple question may help the patient to envision the benefits of the health behavioral change: "If you would decide to make this change, where would you be, say in 4 years?" Likewise, looking back at the good times before the health problems may evoke memories of better times, which creates discrepancy with the present situation. To an overweight patient who hardly leaves her home anymore: "You told me that some years ago, you frequently went to the market . . . How . . ." Patient: "Oh yes! I always went with my sister; we walked the complete market, buying some food and stuff, and then went for a coffee at Mr. Chen's. That was beautiful . . . ." The case manager may ask follow-up questions to stimulate the growing enthusiasm of the patient: "What did you buy?" "What coffee did you take? And your sister?" "What was the funniest situation at the market?" This may open the opportunity to explore if and how the patient and her sister can pick up this good old habit again.

Giving Information or Advice

Giving information or advice emphasizes the expert role of the case manager. That does not mean that there is no place for information and advice in MI, but to optimize the effect it can be best employed in an MI way. Berger and Villaume (2013) stress that, while in the field of addiction, the patient has no doubt about the harmful effect of alcohol dependency; in health care, often patients need information to make sense of the need for behavioral change. Patients make sense with the information as they understand or have understood it, whether the information was complete and correct or not. Giving correct information in a way that the patient is willing and able to accept that information may be key to behavioral change for many patients.

The sting is in delivering the information itself. First of all, there is an important relational component which may be overlooked in health care situations. Information is much better received and accepted if the patient trusts the case manager. As a consequence, the first concern of the case manager is building rapport with the patient. Patients start trusting a case manager if the case manager listens to them, understands their concerns, and values them as unique persons and as experts in their own lives. This refers to the spirit of MI. Second, patients explain their current behavior based on practical reasoning by which their explanation makes perfect sense to themselves. When a case manager responds through correcting obvious flaws in the patient's reasoning, the case manager confronts the patient by questioning his or her competence. And by telling the patient he or she "must take the medication" or "ought to stop buying so many cigarettes," the case manager confronts the patient by questioning his or her autonomy (Berger & Villaume, 2013).

In MI, confront is a "don't," so Berger and Villaume suggest another approach. The quintessence is influencing the patient's sense making in such a way that the patient experiences oneself as altering the sense making. By this, the case manager affirms both patient competence and autonomy. First, the case manager needs to understand the current sense making of the patient. This can be done by taking time to listen to the patient. Consider this patient's explanation a few months after his myocardial infarction:

> Patient: "I'm on a lot of medication for that now, so no more exercise and I'm glad I still can allow myself my favorite food," followed by a list of unhealthy foods.

> The case manager reacts by reflecting the patient's sense making: "So, because you're taking medication, you're wondering why you should keep exercising and deny yourself pastry on a daily basis."

> The patient will probably confirm the reflection, and next the case manager asks permission to give information: "That's a good question; is it okay if I share some information on that, and then you tell me your thoughts?" The case manager reframes the patient's reasoning in "a good question," and affirms the patient's autonomy by asking permission and by inviting the patient to react on the meaning of the new information for his sense making.

Patient: "Yeah, that's okay."

Case manager: "You're right that medication is very important in preventing a second myocardial infarction. On top of that, the combination of diet and exercise halves your risk of a repeated event. What do you think?"

Patient: "You mean medication is only half of the work? I have to do the other half?"

Case manager: "Yes, the job is best done if you and your medication work together."

Patient: "I'll have to think it over. Is it okay if I come back on that?"

Case manager: "Sure."

The case manager first affirms the patient's opinion on the importance of medication. In this way, the case manager also affirms the patient's competence, which promotes the patient's receptivity for new information. Next, the case manager delivers short, targeted information, tailored to the patient's information needs. Finally, the case manager invites the patient to use the new information to assimilate it in his reasoning and alter his sense making. The patient reaction also gives the case manager the opportunity to learn about the patient's interpretation of the new information. The patient feels respected, listened to, and taken seriously, instead of being told what is wrong about his thoughts and being told what to do.

Change Plan

When the patient is willing to change his or her health behavior, the case manager may address the question of how to change. This refers to the perceived self-efficacy of the patient. Some patients may not want to draft a change plan, and in those cases, it is best not to push through because it may decrease the motivation of the patient. In all other cases, a small, concrete change plan increases the chance of a successful behavioral change. Patients may also feel ambivalent over their ability to change. It is therefore important that the change plan is the patient's change plan, not the case manager's. A first evocative question might be: "What would be the first step?" The change plan consists of both an action planning and a coping planning, the latter directed at coping with potential barriers and setbacks. In composing the change plan, the case manager also discusses potential resources with the patient: persons who may help or support the patient making this change, tools available, apps, or websites. Finally, goals of the change plan, expressed in terms of: "How do I see that this plan works?" are also part of the small change plan.

Discord and Resistance

Miller and Rollnick (2013) stress that the concept "resistance" seems to hold the patient responsible for tension, difficulties, and disagreements in the conversation. However, in a conversation, there are two parties involved, and "resistance" refers to tension in the relationship between these two parties. But this concept labels the patient. The concept "discord" is a better description of the phenomenon: something is happening between two persons, and this something hinders the constructive conversation about behavioral change.

Discord is not the same as sustain talk. Through sustain talk, the patient communicates his or her autonomous choice not to change, or expresses one side of the ambivalence about change. So, sustain talk is about the target behavior. Discord is about the relationship, and is observable through signs like disengagement from the conversation, opposition ("It is easy for you to say; I'm the one who has to take these pills"; "You can't tell me what to do."), and defending ("I'm not responsible."). In case of discord, the case manager should take a step back and reconsider his or her approach, maybe going too fast for the patient, or threatening the patient's autonomy. If the first is the case, the case manager can acknowledge the patient's position and reflect the ambivalence: "That is true; talking about it is much easier than actually taking these pills. Especially when these pills have both positive effects and side effects." If the patient's autonomy is at issue, the case manager should emphasize the patient's control: "You're right, I can't tell you what to do; you are the person who decides." Discord is best prevented and restored through the spirit of MI.

In their focus of MI in health care practice, Berger and Villaume (2013) use the terms "issue resistance" and "relational resistance." Issue resistance is the type of sustain talk that derives from the patient's explanatory model for his or her health problem and health behavior connected to the explanatory model: "I can't cut down on beer now, way too much stress!" So, issue resistance is an important subject to address, but it should be done in an MI way, through the spirit of MI. Relational resistance arises from the case manager's reaction to the patient's issue resistance, and resembles the concept of "discord."

Shared Decision Making

Shared decision making (SDM) can be defined as "a process by which a health care choice is made by the patient (or significant others, or both) together with one or more health care professionals" (Légaré et al., 2014, p. 7). Like MI, SDM is an example of patient-centered care practice. The importance of SDM is located in both ethical principles and considerations about efficiency and effectiveness.

Patient involvement and participation is an ethical right, and through the SDM process the patient is well informed about health conditions, health problems, and options. Moreover, SDM involves patient participation in the decision making. Thus, SDM derives from the core value of individual self-determination and autonomy (Elwyn et al., 2012).

Patient involvement through the process of SDM may also enhance patient participation in the execution of the chosen interventions. When "what matters most to the patient" (Elwyn et al., 2012, p. 1361) has been an important focus of the decision-making process, and if the patient agrees to a certain health regimen including taking medication and lifestyle change, this increases the chance of the patient's acceptance of the health regimen.

Both SDM and MI are solidly based on a good and trusting working relationship between patient and case manager. Besides, applying SDM and MI requires good clinical communication skills.

The Method of SDM

There are different SDM models; in the following, we combine two of them (Elwyn et al., 2012; Légeré et al., 2014). Practicing SDM, however, demands flexibility. The case manager should always tailor the steps to the patient's needs and health literacy.

Health Problem

The first step is to define and explain the health problem to the patient. To this end, the case manager links information to what the patient already knows. When listening to the patient sharing what he or she already knows, the case manager may also observe misconceptions, which may influence the patient's preferences.

Decision to Be Made

In this step, the case manager and the patient establish the subject(s) about which decision(s) have to be made. Elwyn et al. (2012) add "choice talk" to this step, meaning making patients aware that various options exist.

Present Options

To avoid jumping to conclusions, it may be sensible to first list the options and next (if necessary) provide information about the options.

Effectively giving information means information in small amounts, and targeted to the patient's needs. After giving information, check the patient's reaction and sense making. Relevant information comprises benefits, risks, and costs. Limit the options to the realistic ones: those that are feasible and effective.

Depending on the decision, the options, and the patient, the case manager may provide the patient with nonverbal information, such as reliable websites, information leaflets, a DVD. At this point, or any other point in the decision-making process, the patient may need more time to think things over, or to discuss options with other persons.

Values and Preferences

The question "What matters most to you?" is an important question in the SDM process. The case manager can support the patient by exploring the effects of the decisions on the patient's values: "How would this decision (or this option) affect your . . . (family, work, social life)?"

Self-Efficacy

Discuss the patient's confidence in the ability to perform his part of the options, and to accept possible burden or harm as a result of the options.

Summarize

Summarize the options and the content of the discussion between the patient and the case manager per option. If appropriate, the case manager may make a recommendation.

Moving to a Decision

Check if the patient is ready to make a decision. Some patients may need more time, more information, or want to discuss the decision with other persons. In this situation, the decision will be deferred.

In many health care decisions, the patient's preference is a component in the health care decision. The actual choice is a shared decision, made in close cooperation with significant others and health care professionals.

NOTE

[1] Thanks to Irma Stijnman for these beautiful personalized goals.

REFERENCES

Allison, J., Bes, R., & Rose, G. (2012). Motivational Interviewing Target Scheme. MITS 2.1. An instrument for practitioners, trainers, coaches and researchers. Explanation & guidance. Retrieved from http://www.motivationalinterviewing.org/sites/default/files/MITS_2.1.pdf

Apodaca, T. R., Jackson, K. M., Borsari, B., Magill, M., Longabaugh, R., Mastroleo, N. R., & Barnett, N. P. (2016). Which individual therapist behaviors elicit client change talk and sustain talk in motivational interviewing? *Journal of Substance Abuse Treatment, 61*, 60–65. doi:10.1016/j.jsat.2015.09.001

Bem, D. J. (1967). Self-perception: An alternative interpretation of cognitive dissonance phenomena. *Psychological Review, 74*(3), 183–200. doi:10.1037/h0024835

Berger, B. A., & Bertram, C. T. (2015). Motivational interviewing and specialty pharmacy. *Journal of Managed Care & Specialty Pharmacy, 21*(1), 13–17. doi:10.18553/jmcp.2015.21.1.13

Berger, B. A., & Villaume, W. A. (2013). *Motivational interviewing for health care professionals: A sensible approach.* Washington, DC: American Pharmacists Association. ISBN: 9781582121802

Chow, C. K., Jolly, S., Rao-Melacini, P., Fox, K. A. A., Anand, S. S., & Yusuf, S. (2010). Association of diet, exercise, and smoking modification with the risk of early cardiovascular events after acute coronary syndromes. *Circulation, 121*, 750–758. doi:10.1161/CIRCULATIONAHA.109.891523

Elwyn, G., Frosch, D., Thomson, R., Joseph-Williams, N., Lloyd, A., Kinnersley, P., . . . Barry, M. (2012). Shared decision making: A model for clinical practice. *Journal of General Internal Medicine, 27*(10), 1361–1367. doi:10.1007/s11606-012-2077-6

Jorstad, H. T., von Birgelen, C., Alings, A. M. W., Liem, A., van Dantzig, J. M., Jaarsma, W., . . . Peters, R. J. G. (2013). Effect of a nurse-coordinated prevention programme on cardiovascular risk after an acute cardiovascular syndrome: Main results of the RESPONSE randomised trial. *Heart, 99*, 1421–1430. doi:10.1136/heartjnl-2013-303989

Légaré, F., Stacey, D., Turcotte, S., Cossi, M.-J., Kryworuchko, J., Graham, I. D., . . . Donner-Banzhoff, N. (2014). Interventions for improving the adoption of shared decision making by healthcare professionals. *Cochrane Database of Systematic Reviews, (9)*, CD006732. doi:10.1002/14651858.CD006732.pub3

Lundahl, B., Moleni, T., Burke, B. L., Butters, R., Tollefson, D., Butler, C., & Rollnick, S. (2013). Motivational interviewing in medical care settings: A systematic review and meta-analysis of randomized controlled trials. *Patient Education and Counseling, 93*, 157–168. doi:10.1016/j.pec.2013.07.012

Miller, W. R., & Rollnick, S. (2002). *Motivational interviewing: Preparing people for change* (2nd ed.). New York, NY: Guilford Press. ISBN: 9781572305632

Miller, W. R., & Rollnick, S. (2013). *Motivational interviewing: Helping people change* (3rd ed.). New York, NY: Guilford Press. ISBN: 9781609182274

Rollnick, S., Miller, W. R., & Butler, C. C. (2007). *Motivational interviewing in health care: Helping patients change behavior.* New York, NY: Guilford Press. ISBN: 9781593856120

PART IV

Transitions of Care and Accreditation Care in Integrated Case Management

CHAPTER 9

Interdisciplinary Care Teams Fostering Successful Transitions of Care

Kathleen Fraser
Rebecca Perez

To truly achieve whole person care that integrates medical and psychosocial aspects of an individual, case managers that can support addressing health behaviors as well as behavioral health are among the most important resources in healthcare.

—Paul Ciechanowski

OBJECTIVES

- Define interdisciplinary care team concepts for integrated case management
- Know the key elements in creating and maintaining the interdisciplinary teams
- Understand the role of the patient navigators, extenders, or health coaches
- Understand critical elements for improving transitions of care for patients
- Know the successful skill set of the integrated case manager, to impact successful transitions of care for medically complex patients
- Understand the various case management practice settings and genres
- Discuss the emerging focus of population health

Interdisciplinary Team Concepts

Interdisciplinary teams are increasingly prevalent and are central to health care reform. Blinders, silos, and territories impede the case manager's view of the full health care system. What can case managers do to create change for their patients and become true integrated case managers? The foundation of integrated care is a holistic view of the individual and personal health as complex, integrated systems, rather than a simple sum of independent body systems. It follows that integrated care begins with an assessment of patients for conditions and or the risk of developing conditions in addition to the ones they present. To do so effectively, the case manager must assemble a health care team. Teams should focus on a defined goal with parameters, such as a specific unaddressed care need, improvement on a quality measure, a setting, or a patient population. Remember your team members come from diverse training and backgrounds within the same specialty. Teams must develop respect, competence, accountability, and trust for each other to define and treat not only patient problems but those affecting process and workflow. Together, team members will determine the team's mission and common goals. The outcomes of the team's work must be deemed superior to individually based outcomes.

Collaborative Partnership Approach to Care

Research suggests that high functioning interdisciplinary teams share a set of characteristics, including, but not limited to, positive leadership, a supportive team climate, clarity of vision, appropriate skill mix, and respect and understanding of all roles. A team should have a shared mission using improved clinical systems to deliver improved care to a patient population supported by operational and financial systems. Such care is continuously evaluated through improvement processes and effectiveness measurement (Agency for Healthcare Research and Quality, 2015). Creating the collaborative team among physicians, pharmacists, nurses, case managers, social workers, allied health and supporting staff such as claims adjuster or patient's employer, if applicable, is critical to achieving the goals of the team, the organization, and changing the way we deliver health care today. Collaborate and advocate with all stakeholders to develop a care plan across the care continuum. As the health care environment focuses on becoming more cost-effective and efficient, it is important for all disciplines to work as a team in order to:

- Understand the role of each discipline
- Encourage effective communication
- Prevent duplication of services
- Ensure continuity of care

It is key to develop a communication process that defines how the team will solve differences and build collaboration. Position yourself as eyes and ears of physicians, as collaborators in providing good care, assisting with providing information and education. Shift from reliance on abstract principles to using past concrete experiences to guide actions. Shift in perception of situations from separate pieces to whole parts with the ability to recognize what is most relevant. Pass from being a detached observer to an involved performer—actively engaged and fully participating. The integrated case manager should spend less time giving advice, and more time asking questions of the team.

There is no question that industry movement toward integrated health systems, population health management, and value-based reimbursement requires an inter professional approach to care coordination using collaborative care teams. Professional integrated case managers are key members of this new team culture in which trust, respect, and multidisciplinary interdependence are required to achieve effective patient outcomes. Each member of the collaborative care team—whether licensed or unlicensed, clinical or nonclinical—has an important role in care coordination. The key is to verify that all members of the team are crystal clear on their roles, accountabilities, and scope of practice. The interdisciplinary team members should be complexity and relationship focused and serve as resources to each other. This includes making sure that the role and functions of the professional case manager are not inappropriately delegated to unqualified team members.

Non-Licensed Patient Navigator, Extender, or Health Coach

The professional case manager makes a profound difference in his or her patient's life. For many years, the patient's outcomes, although positive, were not always recognized as a direct result of the case manager's plan and intervention. Ironically, as the value of case managers becomes visible, the scarcity of professional case managers is notable. The case manager is needed for chronic illness management, high-risk case management, and integrated case management (ICM). Because of the demand, many organizations are assembling a partnership with a non-licensed patient navigator, health coach, patient extender, or other organizational titles, to assist in the care coordination of patients. The professional case manager directs a patient-centered model utilizing patient navigators to reduce barriers to care. The navigators support individual patients through the health care continuum as it pertains to their specific disease, ensuring that barriers to care are resolved and that each stage of care is as easy for the patient as possible (Thomas & Moore, 2012).

The concept of patient navigation is about providing education and emotional support to patients and guiding them through the health care maze under the direction of the professional case manager. The patient navigator benefits not only patients, but also hospital systems and insurance companies. The navigator supports the patient-centered care plan created by the professional case manager, in collaboration with the case manager, patient, and other appropriate partners. The navigator program follows the Case Management Society of America Standards of Practice and is outcome driven. Health care systems and payers expect positive patient-centered outcomes. The common metrics used to measure outcomes are improved patient and caregiver satisfaction, improved quality, reduced costs, and optimized resources and revenue. Patient navigators work in a variety of settings including communities, hospitals, homes, primary care offices, and tertiary care. The navigators do not require formal clinical training, license, or certification; however, these would be beneficial. It is essential that navigators collaborate with licensed and certified professional case managers to supplement, complement, and assist patients/clients through the health care system. They should never be used as a substitute for the professional case manager. Navigators are trained by the professional case manager to recognize potential roadblocks to services.

More than 40 million Americans are 65 years of age or older. The number of Americans in this age bracket will double by 2030 to almost 20% of the population. Most have one chronic disease and at least a fourth have two or more. Due to global factors, it is likely the older demographic will be poorer, increasing the risk of disease and disability. In the space of 2 years, 2000 to 2002, a Medicare beneficiary could conceivably see up to 16 physicians over a year. This excludes pharmacists, lab and imaging technicians, and other subspecialists (Cosgrove, 2015). Treatment of chronic illnesses now accounts for almost 93% of Medicare spending. Medicare fee for service program spent an average of $32,658 per beneficiary with six or more chronic conditions compared to an average of $9,738 for all other beneficiaries (Hatch, Isakson, Wyden, & Warner, 2015). The focus here is patient safety and self-management. The navigator (which includes community health workers, health coaches, et al.) assists the integrated case manager to work at the top of their license by being a true extension of the case manager interacting with the patient only when directed by the case manager and agreed upon by the patient.

Transitions of Care

Transitions of care is the movement of patients from one health care practitioner, level of care, and/or a different setting to another, as their condition and care need change. For successful transitions of care, use your critical thinking skills, using a holistic approach, knowing your research which, in turn, makes the arguable inarguable. Focus on communicating any changes to the health care team, which improves outcomes for our patients, especially those with complex injuries or diagnosis.

Integrated Case Manager Skills Required for Successful Transitions of Care

- The ability to coordinate medical and behavioral interventions
- Professional, yet empathic demeanor
- Focus on patient-centered autonomy and assisting the patient in defining goals
- The ability to bring patients into a collaborative partnership with meaningful communication with patient, family, care team, employer, and claims professional
- The ability to not only engage stakeholders but turn that engagement into activation

Activation is an integral part of the transition process. This involves the talent of the case manager to instill the knowledge, skills, confidence, and resources to patients to manage their disease state in an active and informed manner. A patient-centered approach meets patients at their personal level of readiness to learn and accomplish their health-related goals. Focus is on patient–provider shared decision making in all phases of their treatment. Patients with the highest levels of activation display interest, involvement, and actively decide the best course of involvement for themselves. In addition, high activation levels are associated with decreased health care costs as well. The case manager coordinates cost-effective plans, providing high-quality continuous care that eliminates duplication of services and wasted benefit dollars. These are often dollars which can be hard to track but occur when there is one case manager from beginning to fruition! Fraction of care can be avoided by fewer case manager handoffs. The role of the case manager is to communicate with clients and providers to reassess, educate, and develop a care or treatment plan. Most importantly, the case manager is to promote self-efficacy and engage patients in their treatment protocol.

The case manager is responsible for facilitation and coordination of care for the client while communicating with the interprofessional care team, involving the client in the decision-making process to minimize fragmentation in the services provided, and preventing risk for unsafe care and suboptimal outcomes. To facilitate effective and competent performance, the professional case manager should demonstrate knowledge of health insurance and funding sources, health care services, human behavior dynamics, health care delivery and financing systems, community resources, ethical and evidence-based practice, applicable laws and regulations, clinical standards and outcomes, and health information technology and digital media relevant to case management practice. The skills and knowledge base of a case manager may be applied to individual clients such as in the hospital setting, or to groups of clients such as in disease, chronic care, or population health management models. Often case managers execute their responsibilities across settings, providers, over time, and beyond the boundaries of a single episode of care. They also employ the use of health and information technology and tools. Successful interdisciplinary teams are able to improve the client/patient care experience and outcomes by increasing the coordination of services, integrating health care for the patient's wide range of health needs, empowering patients/clients as active partners in care, and empowering clients to problem-solve by exploring options of care, when available, and alternative plans, when necessary, to achieve desired outcomes.

Doctors, nurses, and other health care professionals remain the most trusted sources for health information, according to a 2010 Pew Internet and American Life Project and a 2012 Deloitte Study (Fox, 2012; World of DTC Marketing, 2012). However, online sources are becoming a trusted source for specific disease and treatment information. Of the 74% of adults using the Internet, 80% searched for this specific information (Fox, 2012). Social networks are increasing in popularity; however, they are not a regularly used source of health information. The most trusted sites for health-specific information are those that focus on health, like WebMD or Mayo Clinic. Caregivers are found to use social networks to follow others' health updates and are seen as a source of encouragement and support (Fox, 2012). One in four Internet users have reviewed online information about prescription drugs or condition-specific treatments, but are less likely to access the sites of pharmaceutical manufacturers (World of DTC Marketing, 2012). Recommendations for an accurate diagnosis, information about prescription drugs, alternative treatments, recommendations for a physician or specialist, and recommendations for a hospital or other medical facility are sought from health care professionals. Emotional support for a health condition or a quick recommendation related to a health issue are sought from non-health care professionals.

Communication and Transitions of Care

As discussed in Chapter 8, the communication between the patient and the health care team must be continuous and the professional case manager facilitates this communication. The Centers for Medicare and Medicaid have attached financial penalties for health care systems experiencing unnecessary readmissions. Ineffective communication between and among health care providers and patients is a leading cause of medical errors and patient harm. As reported to the Joint

Commission, communication failure is the root cause of these errors and subsequent readmissions (Kwan, Morgan, Stewart, & Bell, 2015). In addition to the added complexities of the new and emerging health care system, only 12% of adults in the United States have the health literacy skills needed to manage the demands of the system, and even these individuals' ability to absorb and use health information can be compromised by stress or illness (Sarkar, Schillinger, & Aronson, 2015).

Barriers to Effective Communication

How well we communicate is determined not by how well we say things but how well we are understood.

—Andree Grove, *Co-founder of Intel*

Hospitals are stressful environments for patients and their families, which can add to confusion, anger, frustration, and errors. This can all lead to fragmented care, unsafe discharges, transition of care failures with less than desirable outcomes with increased costs.

Reflective listening is the key to this work. Listen carefully to your patients/clients. They will tell you what has worked and what has not, what moved them forward and shifted them backward. Whenever you are in doubt about what to do, listen—but listening is essential for effectiveness (Figure 9.1). Forty percent to 80% of the information patients

FIGURE 9.1 Communication of the message.

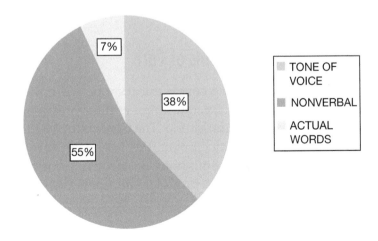

hear in a consultation is lost almost immediately. Seventy percent of patients leave the hospital without understanding their treatment. Affirm patient/caregiver dignity and respect cultural, religious, socioeconomic, and sexual diversity. Assess cultural values and beliefs, including perceptions of illness, disability, and death. Use the patient/caregiver's values and beliefs to strengthen the support system and understand traditions and values as they relate to health care and decision making.

The Integrated Case Manager Role in Education

Education by the integrated case manager is critical for transitions of care, insuring the patient is knowledgeable about and is adhering to the treatment plans prescribed, such as medication regimen or therapy not initiated in the hospital. Notify the treating physician of any discrepancies, inconsistencies, or misunderstandings and provide educational information to support patient/caregivers' participation in the plan of care. Simplify when possible to ensure that patients understand their risks if they do not adhere to medication regimens. Ask patients about the consequences of not taking their medications or treatment guidelines. Have patients restate the positive benefits of taking their medications and following treatment orders. Address fears and concerns to assist individuals in transitions, develop and identify self-management tools, and provide them with the resources for and links to support.

Whenever possible, facilitate self-determination and self-care through the tenets of advocacy, shared decision making, and education. Turn the passenger into a driver while assisting the client in the safe transitioning of care to the next most appropriate level, setting, and/or provider.

Seven tips for clinicians
- Use plain language
- Limit information (3–5 key points)
- Be specific and concrete, not general
- Demonstrate, draw pictures, use models
- Repeat/summarize
- Teach-back (confirm understanding)
- Be positive, hopeful, empowering

CASE STUDY

The following case study highlights how select ICM tools are used for safe transitions of care by the case manager and the interdisciplinary team, for an individual in an acute care facility following an exacerbation of his emphysema. The case illustrates how the team can determine educational needs and develop and support the plan of care. Each aspect of the treatment plan requires an assessment of the patient's knowledge and motivation.

A 63-year-old White male presents to the emergency room with complaints of shortness of breath (SOB) upon exertion as well as at rest. He shows signs and symptoms of a lung infection–productive cough, greenish-yellow sputum, increased dyspnea, tachycardia, fever, and weight loss. He was diagnosed with emphysema at age 53.

Vitals
- RR: 32
- Blood pressure: 160/95 mmHg
- Pulse: 160
- Weight: 150 pounds, Ht: 6'0"
- Temp: 101.8°F

Diagnoses
- Atrial fibrillation
- Depression
- Emphysema

Past surgical history
- None

Previous inpatient hospitalizations
- No other hospitalizations until now. States that daughter being a nurse helps to keep him out of the hospital.

Current medications
- Escitalopram 10 mg once daily for depression
- Diltiazem ER 240 mg once daily for atrial fibrillation
- Long-acting beta agonist
- Long-acting anticholinergic

Economic/income status
- Monthly social security income: $694
- Monthly Veterans Administration (VA) income: $795

Payor sources
- Medicare Health Maintenance Organization (HMO) policy
- VA benefits

Social history
- Smoker for 35 years; ceased upon emphysema diagnosis at age 53
- Averages two to three alcohol drinks per week
- Divorced for 24 years, one adult daughter who is a registered nurse (RN)
- Part-time employment as a teacher for after-school children in ex-wife's daycare; had to take early retirement from teaching in the public school system because of decreased stamina and SOB

Based on presenting symptoms, the emergency physician admitted him to the hospital with a primary diagnosis of emphysema with exacerbation. Admitting orders and projected length of stay (LOS):

- 4-day LOS
- Chest x-ray indicative of emphysema (obvious bullous disease)
- Sputum culture positive for pneumococcus
- Pulmonary consult—patient considered GOLD category D on combined assessment (based on current hospitalization for exacerbation)
- Post-bronchodilator spirometric results
- $FEV_1/FVC = 60\%$, $FEV_1 = 50\%$ of predicted value for age, sex, and size
- Oximetry testing
- Oxygen saturation = 89%
- Ambulatory for short distances due to SOB
- Continent of bladder and bowel

Actual hospitalization LOS: 10 days. Patient no longer ambulatory, now bedbound and periods of bladder and bowel incontinence. Requires bedpan. Methicillin-resistant staphylococcus aureus (MRSA) infected lungs requiring IV vancomycin. The patient received the following instructions on discharge:

- Outpatient pulmonary rehabilitation referral
- Outpatient physical therapy
- Referral to local chronic obstructive pulmonary disease (COPD) support group
- New medications: systemic corticosteroids, IV antibiotic, inhaled corticosteroids

- Continue with oxygen concentrator and portable oxygen system, as needed
- Nutritional consult for weight gain
- Influenza and pneumococcal immunization
- Home health referral for case management, physical therapy, nurse aide, and nursing
- Follow-up with pulmonologist in 2 weeks for evaluation and treatment plan

Barriers

Holiday weekend (New Year's Eve discharge day and next day NYD)

IV vancomycin

Medicare HMO refused more days in hospital, skilled nursing facility (SNF), or nurse aide assistance

Daughter lives 3 hours from patient, works full time with three children in elementary school. Son-in-law works full-time day job as well. Patient refusing to move in with daughter when he is a burden. Daughter welcomes him to move in but patient still refuses until he is stronger. ■ ■ ■

Case Management Intake and Assessment

The case manager should complete an assessment using their organization's assessment tool and incorporating the ICM assessment tools. The patient is a college graduate and was a teacher, but education does not always translate to health literacy. Unless an individual is a health care professional, there is still rationale to administer the REALM-R to determine health literacy level. The patient refused because stated "my daughter is an RN; she can take care of me." Upon discharge, his level of mobility declined to bed-bound status. Daughter has taken vacation to stay in her father's home to be with patient during hospital stay.

Individuals with a recent transition in care are at risk for medication errors. Case managers can refer to the discharge medication reconciliation and confirm that the patient and/or caregivers understand any changes. This patient has a history of medication nonadherence due to financial issues. He receives monthly VA income but has never accessed any VA health benefits. He states he has regular insurance and does not want to deplete VA funds.

Medication Assessment

The medication assessment should cover the prescribed medications and include the patient's knowledge of the following:

- Does patient know the name of the medication?
- What is the dosage of the medication, and how often is it to be used?
- Does the patient understand the purpose of the medication?
  - Why is he using it? What is it supposed to do for his condition?
  - What are the things he should watch for to determine if the medication is working?
- What are some of the adverse effects he may see, and what should he do if he experiences them? Are there things he can do to minimize any adverse effects? When should he contact his physician?
- How long does he have to continue to take the medication?
- How often does the medication need to be refilled? With his inhalers, does he know how to judge when a refill is needed? When is the next refill due? Where will the patient get the next refill?

Although these steps are listed sequentially in this example, opportunities may present themselves at other times in conversation with the patient. For example, if the patient expresses resistance while reviewing any of the medications, this may be an opportunity to explore the source of that resistance.

The diagnosis of depression is likely to undermine some of the patient's confidence in his ability to cope with the rehabilitation demands and follow the care plan (Katon et al., 2012). It is recommended that the case manager go beyond assessing his understanding of the importance of making the changes needed and his willingness to make those changes and adhere to the plan. It is important to assess his confidence as well. He may know he needs to change and why. He may even be willing to change. However, if he is not confident that he can change, his chances of success will diminish. "There are certainly a lot of things you are going to be doing to manage your health. If I were to ask you how confident you are that you can do the things we've discussed on a scale from 1 to 10, where 1 means there is no way you can do it and 10 means you have no doubt you can do it, where would you rate yourself?"

As with willingness and importance, the case manager would respond so as to elicit additional information. For example, if the patient rates himself a 2, the case manager may ask why he did not rate himself a 10, or what would it take for him to get to a 10. Questions such as these may elicit the patient's view of his own strengths and any barriers he sees to his success. The case manager can then use this information to do additional questioning and provide more specific and relevant information. The desired outcome is that the ICM will have an "adherence temperature." Are they cold in their readiness, perception of importance, and confidence, or are they hot to get going? As noted previously, the presence of depression will complicate the case.

Social Support

How does the patient perceive his social support system? He is divorced with a grown daughter, son-in-law, and three young grandchildren and lives 3 hours away. He appears to have not accepted the prognosis of emphysema and verbalizes he will regain strength and be independent soon. Using the readiness ruler, the case manager will be able to assess his satisfaction with the amount of support he receives from his family. Areas where the patient has lower scores could be explored similar to the medication readiness questions. For example, "You rated this question a 2. What would it take to get to a 10?" This allows the case manager to explore the person's support needs while allowing him to share what he needs without revealing details he may not be ready to share. For example, "Well, to be a 10, I would need to see my daughter more often which means moving from the city I grew up in and in which my brother still lives." He does not have to divulge any of his own insecurities until he is ready or willing.

With his divorce, a grown child who lives elsewhere, and the inability to return even to reduce work hours until he regains mobility, this patient is at risk for social isolation. It is important to ensure he has the social support that he needs. If not, the case manager could help him explore some options for meeting those needs. The physician has ordered his referral to a support group. However, he refuses to attend stating he does not need it and that he gets all the support he needs from his daughter.

Based on his depression diagnosis, referral for psychotherapy should also be considered. The assessment grid of his social support network may help him realize the value of a support group in his social support structure. At least the case manager has opened the door by creating a small amount of dissonance with his current level of support.

Case Management Practice Settings

Professional case management practice extends to all health care settings across the continuum of health and human services. This may include the payer, provider, government, employer, community, and client's home environment. The specific roles and responsibilities of professional case managers may vary based on their health discipline background and the environment or care setting in which they practice. The practice varies in degrees of complexity, intensity, urgency, and comprehensiveness based on the following four factors:

1. The context of the care setting, such as wellness and prevention, acute, subacute and rehabilitative, skilled care, or end-of-life

2. The health conditions and needs of the client population(s) served, and the needs of the client's family or family caregivers

3. The reimbursement method applied, such as managed care, workers' compensation, Medicare, or Medicaid

4. The health care professional discipline of the designated case manager, such as but not limited to a registered nurse, social worker, physician, rehabilitation counselor, respiratory therapist, and/or disability manager

The following is a representative list of case management practice settings; however, it is not an exhaustive reflection of where professional case managers exist today. Settings where you will find professional integrated case managers are:

- Hospitals and integrated care delivery systems, including acute care, subacute care, long-term acute care (LTAC) facilities, SNFs, and rehabilitation facilities

- Ambulatory care clinics and community-based organizations, including student or university counseling and health care centers, medical and health homes, primary care practices, and federally qualified health centers

- Corporations
- Schools
- Public health insurance and benefit programs such as Medicare, Medicaid, and state-funded programs
- Private health insurance programs such as workers' compensation, occupational health, catastrophic and disability management, liability, casualty, automotive, accident and health, long-term care insurance, group health insurance, and managed care organizations
- Independent and private case management companies
- Government-sponsored programs such as correctional facilities, military health and VA, and public health
- Provider agencies and community-based facilities such as mental/behavioral health facilities, home health services, ambulatory, and day care facilities
- Geriatric services, including residential, senior centers, assisted living facilities, and continuing care retirement communities
- Long-term care services, including home, skilled, custodial, and community-based programs
- End-of-life, hospice, palliative, and respite care programs
- Physician and medical group practices, patient-centered medical home (PCMH), accountable care organizations (ACOs), and physician hospital organizations (PHOs)
- Life care planning programs
- Population health, wellness and prevention programs, and disease and chronic care management companies (Case Management Society of America, 2016)

Complex Populations and Population Health

The populations that case managers serve vary from those that need episodic interventions to those that will require long-term involvement and comprehensive interventions. Regardless of your practice setting, you will encounter individuals spanning the continuum of care. ICM focuses on the most complex of patients, those who have challenges in the four domains of health, but especially those with both medical and mental illness conditions. Examples of complex populations include but are not limited to:

- Children with special health care needs
- Children in foster care
- Intellectually and developmentally disabled
- Disabled adults
- Elderly with special needs and disabilities
- Long-term support services recipients
- Traumatic brain injury
- Traumatic work-related injuries
- Serious and persistent mental illness

Reimbursement sources for these populations can range from Medicaid, Medicare, Medicare and Medicaid, waiver programs, commercial insurance, injury/disability settlements, and other state-sponsored reimbursement programs for special needs. These populations require and should have aggressive case management and care coordination intervention.

Let us look at two case studies that fit this description and would benefit from an integrated approach.

Traumatic Brain Injury

Parker is a 27-year-old male who suffered a traumatic brain injury 2 years ago because of a motor vehicle accident while he was driving a plumbing van for his employer. Parker was in the intensive care unit (ICU) for 3 weeks on a ventilator due to the injuries sustained in the accident and finally woke from a coma after 3 weeks. He started experiencing seizures a week after waking. Parker's brain injury was isolated to the frontal lobe of his brain. He also suffered multiple fractures and a pneumothorax. Due to his injuries, his acute care stay was 5 weeks long and he was transferred to an acute rehabilitation facility to complete physical and cognitive therapy. He did experience short-term memory loss, word-searching, periods of slow response to conversation, delayed reactions, and poor impulse control. Parker's physical injuries resolved without any residual disability and his seizures were controlled by medication. He was discharged from acute rehab after 4 weeks with recommendations to continue outpatient cognitive therapy.

Prior to the accident, Parker lived with his girlfriend Brandy in a small house outside of Chattanooga, Tennessee. Brandy is his primary social support; Parker's only family connection is a sister who lives 2 hours away. Due to his seizure disorder and need for continued cognitive therapy, his health care team did not clear him to drive. Brandy agreed to take Parker to his outpatient therapy and follow-up appointments. Within 2 weeks of returning home, Brandy observed that Parker became easily agitated and angry, often yelling at her and using foul language. He often forgot to bathe or change clothes. He was unable to finish most tasks he started. Brandy decided to move away from Parker and sever their relationship as his behaviors were too much for her to manage. Parker became very depressed after Brandy left and started walking to town to drink in the local tavern to pass the time. He often forgot to eat, to take his seizure medications, and neglected his hygiene and housekeeping.

His visits to the tavern progressed to daily, with daily intoxication. He often walked home alone and occasionally woke up in the front yard of his house. His drinking escalated and the tavern owner had to call the sheriff because Parker would pass out on the floor of the tavern. The sheriff took Parker to the local community hospital to "dry out" because he did not want to charge Parker or keep him in jail.

This behavior continued until one night after drinking, he had a grand mal seizure. He was transported to the local community hospital and one of the emergency department (ED) nurses decided to call the outpatient rehab facility where Parker was supposed to receiving cognitive rehab to see if he could be assigned a case manager.

Parker will need long-term involvement by case management to help coordinate needed services to address his cognitive deficits and then to make sure he continues to take medication for the seizure disorder. Since Brandy left, Parker has not seen a physician or attended outpatient rehab. He has the financial means to access care and services due to a large monetary settlement after his accident, but lacks the insight, ability, or support to follow through.

Deborah Gutteridge, MS, CBIS, regional director of marketing and development for NeuroRestorative tells us, "Individuals with traumatic brain injury often experience long-term challenges related to dysfunctional behaviors. Brain injuries often impact an individual's ability to control impulses and deductively reason to make safe decisions. They may lack the insight to be able to follow a substance abuse program necessitating the need for continued, post-acute cognitive therapy."

The Substance Abuse and Mental Health Services Administration supports the need for special interventions related to brain injury and substance use:

> *Some brain injuries are associated with decreases in certain brain chemicals, and a patient's use of alcohol may be an attempt to compensate for this deficiency. However, because of the brain injury, these patients may experience stronger effects from smaller amounts of alcohol than they did before the injury. Resumption of use may cause dramatic worsening of memory or other cognitive functions. The National Head Injury Foundation has stated that any level of alcohol or drug use is contraindicated in all patients with traumatic brain injury, not only because alcohol and drug use is a risk factor for reinjury, but also because it significantly exacerbates cognitive deficits in these patients.* (Center for Substance Abuse Treatment, 1995)

Elderly With Special Needs and Disabilities

Evelyn is an 87-year-old woman with coronary artery disease, hypertension, and chronic kidney disease because of hypertension. Up until 1 year ago she lived with her son Jerome who worked nights as a security guard. Jerome was very attentive to his mother and made sure she kept all medical appointments and took her medicine as prescribed. Evelyn was able to cook breakfast and dinner for Jerome, do light housekeeping like dusting and washing dishes. She could perform personal care and accompany Jerome to the grocery store and church on Sunday. Evelyn had many friends at church with whom she would chat by phone during the week. Jerome passed away suddenly a year ago and Evelyn moved in with her daughter Sharon. Over the last year, Evelyn has deteriorated, becoming significantly weak. She can barely perform personal care, has become incontinent of urine, misses many of her medications and medical appointments, and has experienced several falls resulting in ED visits.

When meeting with Evelyn in Sharon's home, she is very quiet and provides only limited answers to questions. Bruises are noted on Evelyn's arms and lower legs. Sharon dominates the conversations by sharing her own medical and mental health concerns. She complains about her mother while Evelyn is in the room, that she is a burden, does not take care of herself, needs to be changed because she wets herself, does not help to cook or clean. Sharon wants her mother moved into a nursing home as soon as possible. When asked about her mother's falls, Sharon just said she's clumsy. The case manager asked Sharon about Evelyn's medicines and medical appointments. Sharon said she was often too sick and nervous to take her mother to the doctor and she could not make her mother take her pills. Evelyn was asked if she was keeping in touch with her friends and she quietly responded, "No."

The change in Evelyn's overall condition cannot be completely related to advancing age, but may be the result of a more serious situation. Evelyn went from a safe and caring environment to one that may be unsafe and is non-supportive. Her falls may be related to increasing weakness, but could also be the result of elder abuse. Evelyn needs urgent interventions to ensure safety. Should that be placement in a facility? Should the case manager work with Sharon to recognize and address her mental health challenges? What are Evelyn's wishes?

Moving Toward Population Management

In recent years, health care leaders, employers, health plan providers, policy makers, and the public have recognized that health care costs continue to increase year after year, and the ability to meet health care needs cannot be

FIGURE 9.2 Institute for Healthcare Improvement Triple Aim.

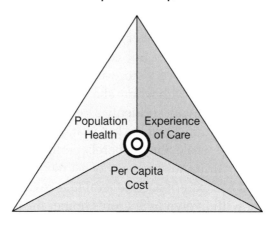

sustained over time (Institute for Healthcare Improvement [IHI], 2009). In the United States, we spend more per capita for health care than any other nation in the world but have overall a less healthy population (IHI, 2009).

In 2007, the IHI asked the question "How do we find ways to drive better value from the resources invested while understanding the complexity and misalignment of our current healthcare system?" IHI's answer to this question was to develop an approach called the "Triple Aim" (Figure 9.2), which will:

- Improve the health of a defined population

- Enhance the patient care experience which includes quality, access, and reliability

- Reduce or at least control the per capita cost of care

The Triple Aim concept has been translated into actions for change:

1. Focus on individuals and families

   a. Use predictive modeling to identify individuals who need intensive services and meet those needs proactively

   b. Customize care plans with input from individuals and their families

2. Redesign primary care and structures

   a. Make appropriate primary care services available around the clock

   b. Use health risk assessments and health coaches to better manage health concerns when they are simple to treat

3. Implement population health management

   a. Partner with communities to share the goal of improved health

   b. Reduce ED visits

   c. Foster connections between public health and health activities

   d. Measure improvement

   e. Develop new spending to support population health

4. Create a cost-control platform

   a. Collaborate with payors to improve care and outcomes for defined populations

   b. Translate the Triple Aim to payment reform models

  c. Base success on quality and patient outcomes

  d. Remove waste in specialty care

5. Integrate systems.

  a. Overcome privacy issues that prevent care coordination between sites and providers of care

  b. Move system level measurement in the right direction (IHI, 2009)

To enhance health, length of life, and reduce illness and disability, we must foster sound advances in science, medicine, public health, and social services (Kaplan, Spittel, & David, 2015). To achieve these objectives, we must better understand the factors that support longer life and reduction in illness and disability. The traditional biomedical model is limited in its ability to foster health and well-being, and focuses strictly on biological processes rather than a goal of helping people live longer and improve quality of life (Kaplan et al., 2015).

According to the National Institutes of Health, a growing body of evidence supports that behavioral and social factors impact at least half of all outcomes, and social factors profoundly impact life expectancy (Kaplan et al., 2015). We all know that people with infections benefit from a quick diagnosis and rapid implementation of treatment, but most of today's burden of illness and disability are associated with chronic conditions and noncommunicable diseases (Kaplan et al., 2015). Heart disease, cancer, and diabetes are common chronic conditions that are expensive to treat and their outcomes are significantly impacted by socioeconomic status and lifestyle. Health behaviors impact both risk and success management. Modification of risk can result in improved outcomes but social factors like income, social support, and access to information can equally affect outcomes.

What Is Population Health Management?

Population health has been discussed for some time and has been defined in the *Journal of Public Health* in 2003 as "the health outcomes of a group of individuals including the distribution of such outcomes within the group" (Kindig & Stoddart, 2003). It is an approach to health that aims to improve the health of an entire human population and has become a significant focus in recent years. A priority of population health is to reduce health inequities or disparities due to social determinants of health (Kaplan et al., 2015).

Let us go back to the Triple Aim for populations. When we speak of populations and population health measures we examine the per capita cost, but within a population may be a subpopulation. Subpopulations are defined by income, race/ethnicity, disease burden, or those served by a particular health system or workforce (Steifel & Nolan, 2012). Triple Aim outcome measures include population health, experience of care, and per capita cost (Steifel & Nolan, 2012; Table 9.1).

The ICM model supports the Triple Aim as well as population health management. Complex patients may be a population or subpopulation of a group. The ICM model addresses medical and behavioral conditions, social factors, access to quality care with the goal of reducing risk for worsening health, improving overall function, and improving quality of life.

TABLE 9.1 Triple Aim Outcome Measures

DIMENSION OF THE TRIPLE AIM	OUTCOME MEASURES
Population health outcomes	• Mortality: years of potential life lost; life expectancy; standardized mortality ratio • Health and functional status: single question assessment; or multidomain assessment • Health life expectancy: combines life expectancy and good health status into a single measure, reflecting years of life in good health • Behavioral and physiologic factors: include blood pressure, BMI, and blood glucose; smoking, alcohol consumption, physical activity, and diet
Experience of care	• Patient surveys • Likelihood to recommend • Key dimensions: safe, effective, timely, efficient, equitable, and patient-centered
Per capita cost	• Cost per member of the population per month • Hospital and emergency department utilization and/or cost

BMI, body mass index.
Source: Steifel and Nolan (2012).

Case managers can play an integral role in helping to achieve the Triple Aim. Our integrated approach to working with patients supports access to appropriate care and services ensuring that an individual receives care for all conditions equally. Complex patients guided to a PCMH, for example, will have enhanced and convenient access to services addressing medical and mental health conditions while being supported in receiving preventative care. In addition to coordinating these consistent and streamlined services, the case manager works to support the patient's decision to make changes that will eventually result in self-management. Synchronization of care with equal attention to medical, behavioral, and social challenges will result in clear economic and quality of life benefits.

REFERENCES

Agency for Healthcare Research and Quality. (2015). AHRQ Health Care Innovations Exchange. Retrieved from https://innovations.ahrq.gov

Case Management Society of America. (2016). *Standards of practice for case management*. Little Rock, AR: Author. Retrieved from http://solutions.cmsa.org/acton/media/10442/standards-of-practice-for-case-management

Center for Substance Abuse Treatment. (1995). Effects of alcohol and other drugs on trauma patients. In *Alcohol and other drug screening of hospitalized trauma patients*. Rockville, MD: Substance Abuse and Mental Health Services Administration (US). Retrieved from https://www.ncbi.nlm.nih.gov/books/NBK64569

Cosgrove, J. (2015). Increasing hospital-physician consolidation highlights need for payment reform. Retrieved from https://www.gao.gov/products/GAO-16-189

Fox, S. (2012). The social life of health information, 2011. Pew Internet & America Life Project. Retreived from http://www.pewinternet.org/2011/05/12/the-social-life-of-health-information-2011

Hatch, O., Isakson, J., Wyden, R., & Warner, M. (2015, May 22). Letter to health care stakeholders. Retrieved from https://www.finance.senate.gov/imo/media/doc/Chronic%20Care%20Working%20Group%20Letter.pdf

Institute for Healthcare Improvement. (2009, January). The Triple Aim: Optimizing health, care and cost. Retrieved from http://www.ihi.org/engage/initiatives/TripleAim/Documents/BeasleyTripleAim_ACHEJan09.pdf

Kaplan, R., Spittel, M., & David, D. (Eds.). (2015). *Population health: Behavioral and social science insights*. Rockville, MD: Agency for Healthcare Research and Quality and Office of Behavioral and Social Sciences Research, National Institutes of Health.

Katon, W., Russo, J., Lin, E. H. B., Schmittdiel, J., Ciechanowski, P., Ludman, E., . . ., Von Korff, M. (2012). Cost-effectiveness of a multicondition collaborative care intervention: A randomized controlled trial. *Archives of General Psychiatry, 69*(5), 506–514. doi:10.1001/archgenpsychiatry.2011.1548

Kindig, D., & Stoddart, G. (2003). "What is population health?" *American Journal of Public Health, 93*, 380–383. doi:10.2105/AJPH.93.3.380

Kwan, J., Morgan, M., Stewart, T., & Bell, C. (2015). Impact of an innovative inpatient patient navigator program on length of stay and 30-day readmission. *Journal of Hospital Medicine, 10*, 799–803. doi:10.1002/jhm.2442

Sarkar, U., Schillinger, D., & Aronson, M. (2015). Literacy and patient care. *UpToDate*, 1–18. Retrieved from http://www.uptodate.com/contents/literacy-and-patient care?topicKey=PC%2F2766&elapse

Steifel, M. M., & Nolan, K. M. (2012). A guide to measuring the Triple Aim: Population health, expereince of care, and per capita cost [IHI Innovation Series white paper]. Cambridge, MA: Institute for Healthcare Improvement. Retrieved from http://www.ihi.org/resources/Pages/IHIWhitePapers/AGuidetoMeasuringTripleAim.aspx

Thomas, E., & Moore, D. (2012). *The emerging field of patient navigation: A golden opportunity to improve healthcare*. Cleveland, OH: The Center for Health Affairs. Retrieved from http://ww1.prweb.com/prfiles/2013/01/02/10285831/12-2012_Patient_Navigation_Publication.pdf

World of DTC Marketing. (2012). Trusted sources of health information. Retrieved from http://worldofdtcmarketing.com/trusted-sources-of-health-information/focus-on-patients

Professional Case Management Accreditation Care Coordination Measures and Outcomes

Kathleen Fraser
Rebecca Perez

Excellence is doing ordinary things extraordinarily well.

—John W. Gardner

OBJECTIVES

- Understand the National Committee for Quality Assurance (NCQA) and the Utilization Review Accreditation Commission (URAC) accreditation with the integrated case management process
- Understand the Nattional Quality Forum (NQF) care coordination measures
- Understand the value demonstrated by an integrated approach

Accreditation is a process of review in which health care organizations participate to demonstrate the ability to meet regulatory requirements and accreditation standards established by a recognized accreditation organization. Care coordination, transitions of care (TOC), patient engagement, and advocacy are core principles for case management. These core principles are measured by accreditation bodies. The benefits of becoming clinically integrated are substantial for improving care delivery, reducing cost, and demonstrating evidence-based outcomes.

Utilization Review Accreditation Commission Case Management Accreditation

Utilization Review Accreditation Commission (URAC) has developed evidence-based measures and standards through inclusive engagement from a range of stakeholders since 1990. Their board of directors is specifically designed to ensure diverse representation from throughout the health care industry. This experience of working with disparate stakeholders is invaluable in today's changing health care environment. To be successful, stakeholders across the health care industry must work together to control costs, raise quality, and improve overall health outcomes.

URAC's case management accreditation standards require companies to establish the policies, procedures, and structure needed for optimal case management performance. These case management standards and performance measures address the increasing demand for excellence in care coordination, including improving consumer engagement, achieving optimal health care outcomes, and managing TOC.

The URAC-accredited case management program:

- Provides collaborative communications between all stake-holders, including patients, family/caregivers, and the health care team
- Develops evidence-based, individualized patient-centered goals to achieve quality health care outcomes
- Ensures that clinical and nonclinical staff have clearly defined roles and responsibilities
- Assesses medical safety, including the need for medical therapy management services
- Uses information support systems to achieve and measure case management performance goals
- Achieves patient self-management goals and optimal levels of wellness through consumer education and engagement
- Ensures safe and effective TOC across settings to prevent poor health outcomes

Organizations that achieve the URAC case management accreditation have an opportunity to obtain the URAC TOC designation. TOC recognizes those organizations making safe care continuity the focus for quality improvements that will be used to reduce errors, preventable readmissions, and poor health outcomes. The coordination of services, education, and the timely transfer of information between hospitals, physicians, post-acute care providers, and patients are essential components of effective TOC management. URAC emphasizes the development of evidence-based, individualized goals that promote quality health care outcomes and ensure that consumers experience safe and effective care transitions across settings. Case management accreditation performance measures have been updated and expanded to include public domain measures focusing in the areas of health outcomes and care transitions, officials say. With an additional designation in TOC, URAC aims to ensure safe and effective patient handoffs through outcome measurements that organizations offer services to handle transitions as they occur, including the timely transfer of information between the appropriate parties.

As an independent, nonprofit organization, URAC has no ties to a specific industry-interest group and no potential conflicts of interest. They are not a member organization or a political advocacy group. Their stated mission is to promote continuous improvement in the quality and efficiency of health care management through accreditation, certification, and measures. Their process facilitates learning in the client's organization, which helps create the framework for continuous improvement. Rather than simply checking off a list of requirements, their approach is non-prescriptive. How an organization meets the accreditation standards can evolve as the processes and systems evolve, to validate commitment to quality and accountability.

Quality Measures for Case Management and Care Coordination

In 2007, the Agency for Healthcare Research and Quality (AHRQ) published a report examining the problems that have led to spiraling health care costs. Based on the key strategy of Care Coordination identified by the Institutes of Medicine, AHRQ developed a working definition of care coordination and frameworks that might predict or explain how care coordination can impact patient outcomes and health care costs (McDonald et al., 2007).

At the time of this report, this was the working definition of Care Coordination developed by AHRQ and it remains unchanged to date:

Care Coordination is the deliberate organization of patient care activities between two or more participants (including the patient) involved in a patient's care to facilitate the appropriate delivery of health care services. Organizing care involves the marshalling of personnel and other resources needed to carry out all required patient care activities, and is often managed by the exchange of information among participants responsible for different aspects of care. (McDonald et al., 2007, p. v)

In this chapter, we examine some of the quality measures related to case management and care coordination. These quality measures are continually evaluated for outcomes and effectiveness. Most case management practice settings are required to participate in quality measures to maintain accreditation. We see this especially in the health plan and insurance company settings. The Centers for Medicare and Medicaid Services also has established quality measures to evaluate quality access to care and services (Centers for Medicare & Medicaid Services, 2016).

An integrated case management (ICM) approach supports most quality measures as our focus in working with a member is to improve access to condition-changing, evidence-based care, movement toward self-management, and improved quality of life. Integrated case managers, through the development of a trusted relationship, will demonstrate improved quality because the patient is more likely to participate in needed care and services.

The National Quality Forum

The National Quality Forum (NQF) was created in 1999 by a coalition of public and private sector leaders to promote and ensure patient protections and health care quality through public reporting of defined measures. The federal government relies on NQF to define measures and health care practices as the best, evidence-based practices to improve care. The federal government, states, and private sector organizations use NQF's endorsed measures to evaluate performance and share information with their stakeholders that include patients and families (NQF, 2017a, 2017b).

For the years 2016 to 2018, NQF defined its strategic direction to: lead, prioritize, and collaborate for better health care measurement by accelerating development of needed measures; identify those measures that should be priority; reduce, select, and endorse measures; drive more

FIGURE 10.1 NQF: Lead. Prioritize. Collaborate.

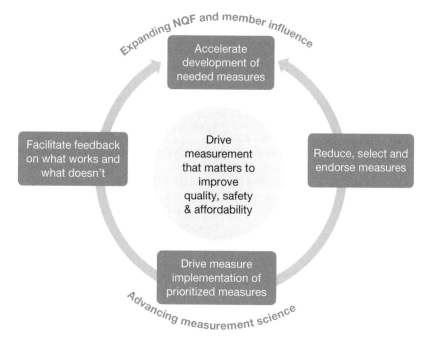

NQF, National Quality Forum.
Source: NQF (2017b).

effective implementation of priority measures; and better understand what works and what does not work (Figure 10.1; NQF, 2017a, 2017b).

Table 10.1 demonstrates the care coordination measures being evaluated by NQF at the time this book was published. NQF continually evaluates the outcomes of these measures and will amend or expand measures to continue efforts to improve quality, safety, and affordability of health care (NQF, 2017a, 2017b):

National Committee for Quality Assurance

The National Committee for Quality Assurance (NCQA) is a not-for-profit, private organization dedicated to improving health care quality. NCQA was founded in 1990 and is the driving force for improvement in our health care system. NCQA strives to elevate health care quality as a priority for the national health care agenda (NCQA, 2017).

TABLE 10.1 NCQA Quality Measures That Impact Case Management

MEASURE	RATIONALE
Advance Care Plan	Advance care planning encompasses communication and discussion regarding treatment preferences that should start before a patient is seriously ill. It provides patients with an opportunity to consider, discuss, and plan their future care with health professionals.
Reconciled Medication List: Reconciled Medication List Received by Discharged Patients (Discharges from an Inpatient Facility to Home/Self Care or Any Other Site of Care)	Percentage of discharges from an inpatient facility (e.g., hospital inpatient or observation, skilled nursing facility, or rehabilitation facility) to home or any other site of care, in which the patient, regardless of age, or their caregiver(s) received a reconciled medication list at the time of discharge including, at a minimum, medications in the specified categories.
Transition Record with Specified Elements Received by Discharged Patients (Discharges from an Inpatient Facility to Home/Self Care or Any Other Site of Care)	Percentage of discharges from an inpatient facility (e.g., hospital inpatient or observation, skilled nursing facility, or rehabilitation facility) to home or any other site of care, in which the patient, regardless of age, or their caregiver(s), received a transition record (and with whom a review of all included information was documented) at the time of discharge including, at a minimum, all of the specified elements.
Timely Transmission of Transition Record (Discharges from an Inpatient Facility to Home/Self Care or Any Other Site of Care)	Percentage of discharges from an inpatient facility (e.g., hospital inpatient or observation, skilled nursing facility, or rehabilitation facility) to home or any other site of care, of patients, regardless of age, for which a transition record was transmitted to the facility or primary physician or other health care professional designated for follow-up care within 24 hours of discharge.
Transition Record with Specified Elements Received by Discharged Patients (Emergency Department Discharges to Ambulatory Care [Home/Self Care] or Home Health Care)	Percentage of discharges from an ED to ambulatory care or home health care, in which the patient, regardless of age, or their caregiver(s), received a transition record at the time of ED discharge including, at a minimum, all of the specified elements.

(continued)

TABLE 10.1 NCQA Quality Measures That Impact Case Management (*continued*)

MEASURE	RATIONALE
Proportion of Children with ED Visits for Asthma with Evidence of Primary Care Connection Before the ED Visit	This measure describes the incidence rate of ED visits for children ages 2–21 who are being managed for identifiable asthma. This measure characterizes care that precedes ED visits for children ages 2–21 who can be identified as having asthma, using the specified definitions. The operational definition of an identifiable asthmatic is a child who has utilized health care services that suggest the health care system has enough information to conclude that the child has an asthma diagnosis that requires ongoing care. Specifically, this measure identifies the use of primary care services and medications prior to ED visits and/or hospitalizations for children with asthma
Percentage of Asthma ED Visits Followed by Evidence of Care Connection	This measure seeks to capture important aspects of follow-up after ED visits for asthma, including prompt follow-up with primary care clinicians and prescription fills for controller medications. This measure characterizes care that follows ED visits with a primary or secondary diagnosis of asthma for children ages 2–21 that occur in the Reporting Year and who are enrolled in the health plan for 2 consecutive months following the ED visit.

ED, emergency department.

Source: NQF (2017b).

NCQA Mission (NCQA, 2017):

"To improve the quality of health care."

NCQA Vision (NCQA, 2017):

"To transform health care quality through measurement, transparency and accountability."

The contributions of NCQA are regularly measured by statistics that track care that is delivered by the nation's health plans. Quality has continued to improve year after year as health protocols have been refined, doctors have changed the way they practice, and patients have become more involved in their care. Many of the measures have resulted in reduction in health care costs and avoided complications. For example, patients who receive beta-blockers after a myocardial infarction reduce their chances of having another heart attack by 40% (NCQA, 2017).

The most widely used set of health care performance measures in the United States is the Healthcare Effectiveness Data and Information Set (HEDIS; NCQA, 2017). HEDIS measures have been in use since the 1990s and have been expanded to include measures for physicians. HEDIS measures impacted by case management are numerous but cover two important categories (NCQA, 2017):

1. Effectiveness of care
2. Accessibility of care

Effectiveness of care measures are extensive; here are a few examples:

- Adult BMI
- Preventative screenings like mammography, cervical cancer, PSA, colonoscopy
- Pharmacotherapy management of COPD
- Controlling high blood pressure
- Comprehensive diabetes care
- Antidepressant medication management

The accessibility of care measures are far less extensive and include:

- Adults' access to preventative/ambulatory health services
- Annual dental visit
- Children with chronic condition
- Initiation and engagement of alcohol and other drug dependence treatment

Organizations strive to meet HEDIS requirements for demonstrating to their stakeholders that quality is a priority.

Organizational Accreditation

Organizational accreditation by NCQA helps organizations meet regulatory requirements and to distinguish themselves from the competition. Accreditation also demonstrates that an organization is committed to quality improvement and value (NCQA, 2017). NCQA provides accreditation to health plans, provider organizations, health plan contractors, and wellness and health promotion organizations. As part of organizational accreditation, NCQA offers accreditation specifically for case management and case management for long-term support services (LTSS) programs.

NCQA case management accreditation directly assesses how case management services are delivered and examines care coordination and quality of care. There is a unique focus on TOC because, as we know, it is in transitions that many complications occur and care coordination may be less than effective.

NCQA recognizes Case Management Society of America's official definition of case management even though various organizations may alter this accepted definition. NCQA requires focus on the core concepts of case management which include assessment, planning, monitoring, and care coordination (NCQA, 2013). In their 2014 Standards and Guidelines for the Accreditation of Case Management Programs, NCQA "continues to promote population health management through accreditation, certification and recognition programs, the addition of a case management accreditation program furthers our goal of improving quality across the continuum of care" (NCQA, 2013). The NCQA Case Management Accreditation Standards appear in Box 10.1.

CM 1: Program Description	The organization describes its case management program, including its evidence base; and reviews and adopts new findings that are relevant to its programs as they become available
CM 2: Patient Identification	The organization identifies and Assessment patients for case management and performs initial assessments
CM 3: Care Planning	The organization has a process to create individual care plans
CM 4: Care Monitoring	The organization has systems in place to support case management activities, and monitors individualized care plans

CM 5: Care Transitions	The organization has a process to manage care transitions, identify problems that could cause care transitions, and prevent unplanned transitions, when possible
CM 6: Measurement and Quality Improvement	The organization measures and works to improve patient satisfaction, program effectiveness, and patient participation
CM 7: Staffing, Training, and Verification	The organization provides training and oversight to its staff, and verifies licensure for staff, as appropriate.
CM 8: Rights and Responsibilities	The organization tells patients what they are entitled to and what is expected of them while they are enrolled in its case management program, and how it handles and resolves complaints
CM 9: Privacy, Security, and Confidentiality Procedures	The organization protects personal health information from inappropriate use, release, or disclosure.
CM 10: Delegation	The organization monitors functions performed by other organizations

Of the ten standards, three standards focus on care coordination:

CM 2: Patient Identification and Assessment

CM 3: Care Planning

CM 4: Care Monitoring

The ICM method supports the achievement of these standards. The ICM assessment and risk tool, the ICM-CAG, comprehensively assesses a patient's needs in the four domains of health to develop a comprehensive care plan that will be monitored over time demonstrating health improvement, or lack of improvement, and why. Case managers will be involved with a patient and assist with any transition of care and update the care plan accordingly. Table 10.2 is a crosswalk to demonstrate the synchronicity of the standards and the ICM method.

TABLE 10.2 CMSA's ICM Methodology Supports NCQA Case Management Elements

STANDARD	DESCRIPTION	ICM MODEL
CM 2; Element A: Population Assessment	1. Assess the characteristics and needs of its patient population and relevant subpopulations	1. The ICM model advocates for organizations to use predictive modeling, assessments, reports, and any other data that points to identifying individuals appropriate for case management interventions with a focus on individuals with health complexity.
CM 2; Elements D and E: Initial Assessment Process and Initial Assessment	1. Initial assessment of a patient's health status, including medical and behavioral condition-specific issues 2. Documentation of clinical history including medications 3. Assessment of ADL 4. Assessment of cognitive issues 5. Assessment of health behaviors 6. Assessment of cultural and linguistic needs 7. Assessment of benefits within the organization	1. Assessment using the ICM-CAG documents all health concerns and treatment for both medical and behavioral conditions and provides an overall risk score. 2. The ICM-CAG covers both medical and behavioral clinical history and treatment, past and present. 3. Functional status is assessed in the biological domain of the ICM-CAG. 4. Past and present cognitive issues are assessed on the Psychological domain. 5. The ability to follow a treatment plan and follow a physician's recommendations is assessed in both the Biological and Psychological domains. 6. Cultural and linguistic needs are assessed in access to the health system. 7. Presence of health care benefits is also assessed in the Health System domain and impact the patient's access to care.

(continued)

TABLE 10.2 CMSA's ICM Methodology Supports NCQA Case Management Elements (*continued*)

STANDARD	DESCRIPTION	ICM MODEL
CM 3; Element A: Care Planning	1. Development of an individualized case management plan with prioritized goals that consider the caregivers' goals, preferences, and desired level of involvement in the case management plan 2. Identification of barriers to meeting goals and complying with the plan	1. The completion of an assessment using the ICM-CAG will result in the ability to prioritize, with the member and caregiver, goals to move toward improved health and function, reduced risk, and self-management. Barriers to achieving goals are also identified and addressed when developing the care plan.
CM 4; Element B: Case Management-Ongoing Case Management	1. Development of an individualized case management plan with prioritized goals that consider the caregivers' goals, preferences, and desired level of involvement in the case management plan 2. Identification of barriers to meeting goals and complying with the plan	1. The development of the care plan as documented in CM 3, Element A, continues with monitoring of case management activities. Reassessment using the ICM-CAG can demonstrate improvement or worsening conditions by comparison of the overall risk score from the initial assessment.

ADL, activities of daily living; CMSA, Case Management Society of America; ICM, Integrated Case Management; ICM-CAG, Integrated Case Management Complexity Assessment Grid; NCQA, National Committee for Quality Assurance.

Source: Reproduced with permission from 2014 Standards and Guidelines for the Accreditation of Case Management Programs by the National Committee for Quality Assurance (NCQA). HEDIS® is a registered trademark of the National Committee for Quality Assurance (NCQA). To purchase copies of this publication, contact NCQA Customer Support at 888-275-7585 or visit www.ncqa.org/publications

Value Demonstrated by an Integrated Approach

The context of the project entailed patients with depression and poorly controlled diabetes mellitus, coronary heart disease, or both, have higher medical complication rates and higher health care costs, suggesting that more effective case management of psychiatric and medical disease might also reduce medical service use and enhance quality of life. This intervention integrated the management of medical and behavioral conditions through proactive follow-up by nurse care managers who were guided by weekly team-based systematic case review that included physicians.

Individualized treatment regimens were guided by treat-to-target principles and applied to achieving improvement in medical and depressive outcomes in depressed patients with out-of-target diabetes, coronary heart disease, or both. Evidence-based behavioral strategies such as motivational enhancement, problem solving, and behavioral activation were used based on a bio-psycho-social assessment of each intervention patient.

In a primary care setting, 214 patients were randomized to the intervention or routine primary care. As compared with controls, patients in the intervention group had greater overall 12-month improvement across glycated hemoglobin levels (difference, 0.58%), LDL cholesterol levels (difference, 6.9 mg/dL), systolic blood pressure (difference, 5.1 mmHg), and SCL-20 depression scores (difference, 0.40 points) ($p <.001$). Patients in the intervention group also were more likely to have one or more adjustments of insulin ($p = .006$), antihypertensive medications ($p <.001$), and antidepressant medications ($p <.001$), and they had better quality of life ($p <.001$) and greater satisfaction with care for diabetes, coronary heart disease, or both ($p <.001$) and with care for depression ($p <.001$).

Without no further intervention after 12 months, the patients were still followed up for 24 months and compared with controls. Intervention patients had a mean of 114 additional depression-free days and lower mean outpatient health costs between $594 and $1,116 per patient. This is a net cost saving, comparing the intervention group versus the usual care group that did not have an integrated nurse case manager. So, even after the $1,204 that the NCM intervention costs over 12 months (the usual care group did not have this cost in year 1), there was a net saving of between $594 and $1,116 in the intervention group at 24 months, compared to the usual care group (Katon et al., 2012).

REFERENCES

Centers for Medicare & Medicaid Services. (2016). Quality measures. Retrieved from https://www.cms.gov/Medicare/Quality-Initiatives -Patient-Assessment-Instruments/QualityMeasures/index.html

Katon, W., Russo, J., Lin, E. H., Schmittdiel, J., Ciechanowski, P., Ludman, E., . . . Von Korff, M. (2012). Cost-effectiveness of a multi-condition collaborative care intervention: A randomized controlled trial. *Archives of General Psychiatry*, *69*(5), 506–514. doi:10.1001/ archgenpsychiatry.2011.1548

McDonald, K. M., Sundaram, V., Bravata, D. M., Lewis, R., Lin, N., Kraft, S., . . . Owens, D. K. (2007). Care coordination. In K. G. Shojania, K. M. McDonald, R. M. Wachter, & D. K. Owens (Eds.), *Closing the quality care gap: A critical analysis of quality improvement strategies* (Vol. 7). Rockville, MD: Agency for Healthcare Research and Quality. Retrieved from https://www.ahrq.gov/sites/default/files/wysiwyg/research/findings/evidence-based-reports/caregap.pdf

National Committee for Quality Assurance. (2013). 2014 CM standards and guidelines. Standards and guidelines for the accreditation of case management programs. Washington, DC: Author.

National Committee for Quality Assurance. (2017). 2017 HEDIS measures. Retrieved from http://www.ncqa.org/Portals/0/HEDISQM/HEDIS2017/HEDIS%202017%20Volume%202%20List%20of%20Measures.pdf?ver=2016-06-27-135433-350

National Quality Forum. (2017a). Care Coordination Endorsement Maintenance Project 2016–2017: Measures. Retrieved from https://www.qualityforum.org/ProjectMeasures.aspx?projectID=83375

National Quality Forum. (2017b). NQF strategic direction 2016–2019. Retrieved from http://www.qualityforum.org/NQF_Strategic_Direction_2016-2019.aspx

CMSA's Definition of Professional Case Management and the Standards of Professional Case Management Practice

2016 Definition of Professional Case Management

Case Management is a collaborative process of assessment, planning, facilitation, care coordination, evaluation and advocacy for options and services to meet an individual's and family's comprehensive health needs through communication and available resources to promote patient safety, quality of care, and cost effective outcomes.

2016 Standards of Professional Case Management Practice

A. Standard: Client Selection Process for Professional Case Management

The professional case manager should screen clients referred for case management services to identify those who are appropriate for, and most likely to benefit from, case management services available within a particular practice setting.

How demonstrated:

- Documentation of consistent use of the client selection process within the organization's policies and procedures.

- Use of screening criteria as appropriate to select a client for inclusion in case management. Examples of screening criteria may include, but are not limited to:

- Barriers to accessing care and services
- Advanced age
- Catastrophic or life-altering conditions
- Chronic, complex, or terminal conditions
- Concerns regarding self-management ability and adherence to health regimens
- Developmental disabilities
- End-of-life or palliative care
- History of abuse or neglect
- History of mental illness, substance use, suicide risk, or crisis intervention
- Financial hardships
- Housing and transportation needs
- Lack of adequate social support including family caregiver support
- Low educational levels
- Low health literacy, reading literacy, or numeracy literacy levels
- Impaired functional status and/or cognitive deficits
- Multiple admissions, readmissions, and emergency department (ED) visits
- Multiple providers delivering care and/or no primary care provider
- Polypharmacy and medication adherence needs
- Poor nutritional status
- Poor pain control
- Presence of actionable gaps in care and services
- Previous home health and durable medical equipment (DME) usage
- Results of established predictive modeling analysis and/or health risk screening tools indicative of need for case management
- Risk-taking behaviors

- Recognition that a professional case manager may receive prescreened client referrals from various sources, including (but not limited to) direct referrals from health care professionals and system-generated flags, alerts, or triggers. In these situations, the case manager should document the referral source and why the client is appropriate for case management services.

B. Standard: Client Assessment

The professional case manager should complete a thorough individualized client-centered assessment that takes into account the unique cultural and linguistic needs of that client including client's family or family caregiver as appropriate.

It is recognized that an assessment:

- Is a process that focuses on evolving client needs identified by the case manager over the duration of the professional relationship and across the transitions of care
- Involves each client and/or the client's family or family caregiver as appropriate
- Is inclusive of the medical, cognitive, behavioral, social, and functional domains, as pertinent to the practice setting the client uses to access care

How demonstrated:

- Documented client assessments using standardized tools, both electronic and written, when appropriate. The assessment may include, but is not limited to, the following components:

   Medical
   - Presenting health status and conditions
   - Medical history including use of prescribed or over-the-counter medications and herbal therapies
   - Relevant treatment history
   - Prognosis
   - Nutritional status

Cognitive and behavioral

- Mental health
  - History of substance use
  - Depression risk screening
  - History of treatment including prescribed or over-the-counter medications and herbal therapies
- Cognitive functioning
  - Language and communication preferences, needs, or limitations
- Client strengths and abilities
  - Self-care and self-management capability
  - Readiness to change
- Client professional and educational focus
  - Vocational and/or educational interests
  - Recreational and leisure pursuits
- Self-management and engagement status
  - Health literacy
  - Health activation level
  - Knowledge of health condition
  - Knowledge of and adherence to plan of care
  - Medication management and adherence
  - Learning and technology capabilities

Social

- Psychosocial status:
  - Family or family caregiver dynamics
  - Caregiver resources: availability and degree of involvement
  - Environmental and residential
- Financial circumstances
- Client beliefs, values, needs, and preferences including cultural and spiritual

- Access to care
  - Health insurance status and availability of health care benefits
  - Health care providers involved in client's care
  - Barriers to getting care and resources
- Safety concerns and needs
  - History of neglect, abuse, violence, or trauma
  - Safety of the living situation
- Advanced directives planning and availability of documentation
- Pertinent legal situations (e.g., custody, marital discord, and immigration status)

Functional

- Client priorities and self-identified care goals
- Functional status
- Transitional or discharge planning needs and services, if applicable
  - Health care services currently or recently received in the home setting
  - Skilled nursing, home health aide, DME, or other relevant services
  - Transportation capability and constraints
  - Follow-up care (e.g., primary care, specialty care, and appointments)
  - Safety and appropriateness of home or residential environment
- Reassessment of the client's condition, response to the case management plan of care and interventions, and progress toward achieving care goals and target outcomes
- Documentation of resource utilization and cost management, provider options, and available health and behavioral care benefits
- Evidence of relevant information and data required for the client's thorough assessment and obtained from multiple sources including, but not limited to:

- Client interviews
- Initial and ongoing assessments and care summaries available in the client's health record and across the transitions of care
- Family caregivers (as appropriate), physicians, providers, and other involved members of the interprofessional health care team
- Past medical records available as appropriate
- Claims and administrative data

C. Standard: Care Needs and Opportunities Identification

The professional case manager should identify the client's care needs or opportunities that would benefit from case management intervention.
How demonstrated:

- Documented agreement among the client, client's family or family caregiver, and other providers and organizations regarding the care needs and opportunities identified
- Documented identification of opportunities for intervention, such as:
  - Lack of established, evidence-based plan of care with specific goals
  - Overutilization or underutilization of services and resources
  - Use of multiple providers and/or agencies
  - Lack of integrated care
  - Use of inappropriate services or level of care
  - Lack of a primary provider or any provider
  - Nonadherence to the case management plan of care (e.g., medication adherence)
    - Low reading level
    - Low health literacy and/or numeracy
    - Low health activation levels
    - Language and communication barriers

- Lack of education or understanding of:
  - Disease process
  - Current condition(s)
  - Medication list
  - Substance use and abuse
  - Social determinants of health
- Lack of ongoing evaluation of the client's limitations in the following aspects of health condition:
  - Medical
  - Cognitive and behavioral
  - Social
  - Functional
- Lack of support from the client's family or family caregiver especially when under stress
- Financial barriers to adherence of the case management plan of care
- Determination of patterns of care or behavior that may be associated with increased severity of condition
- Compromised client safety
- Inappropriate discharge or delay from other levels of care
- High-cost injuries or illnesses
- Complications related to medical, psychosocial, or functional condition or needs
- Frequent transitions between care settings or providers
- Poor or no coordination of care between settings or providers

D. Standard: Planning

The professional case manager, in collaboration with the client, client's family or family caregiver, and other members of the interprofessional health care team, where appropriate, should identify relevant care goals and interventions to manage the client's identified care needs and opportunities. The case manager should also document these in an individualized case management plan of care.

How demonstrated:

- Documented relevant, comprehensive information and data using analysis of assessment findings, client and/or client's family or family caregiver interviews, input from the client's interprofessional health care team, and other methods as needed to develop an individualized case management plan of care

- Documented client and/or client's family or family caregiver participation in the development of the written case management plan of care

- Documented client agreement with the case management plan of care, including agreement with target goals, expected outcomes, and any changes or additions to the plan

- Recognized client's needs, preferences, and desired role in decision making concerning the development of the case management plan of care

- Validated that the case management plan of care is consistent with evidence-based practice, when such guidelines are available and applicable, and that it continues to meet the client's changing needs and health condition

- Established measurable goals and outcome indicators expected to be achieved within specified time frames. These measures could include clinical as well as nonclinical domains of outcomes management: for example, access to care, cost-effectiveness of care, safety and quality of care, and client's experience of care

- Evidence of supplying the client, client's family, or family caregiver with information and resources necessary to make informed decisions

- Promoted awareness of client care goals, outcomes, resources, and services included in the case management plan of care

- Adherence to payer expectations with respect to how often to contact and reevaluate the client, redefine long- or short-term goals, or update the case management plan of care

E. Standard: Monitoring

The professional case manager should employ ongoing assessment with appropriate documentation to measure the client's response to the case management plan of care.

How demonstrated:

- Documented ongoing collaboration with the client, family or family caregiver, providers, and other pertinent stakeholders, so that the client's response to interventions is reviewed and incorporated into the case management plan of care

- Awareness of circumstances necessitating revisions to the case management plan of care, such as changes in the client's condition, lack of response to the case management interventions, change in the client's preferences, transitions across care settings and/or providers, and barriers to care and services

- Evidence that the plan of care continues to be reviewed and is appropriate, understood, accepted by client and/or client's family or family caregiver, and documented

- Ongoing collaboration with the client, family or family caregiver, providers, and other pertinent stakeholders regarding any revisions to the plan of care

F. Standard: Outcomes

The professional case manager, through a thorough individualized client-centered assessment, should maximize the client's health, wellness, safety, physical functioning, adaptation, health knowledge, coping with chronic illness, engagement, and self-management abilities.

How demonstrated:

- Created a case management plan of care based on the thorough individualized client-centered assessment

- Achieved through quality and cost-efficient case management services, client's satisfaction with the experience of care, shared and informed decision making, and engagement in own health and health care

- Evaluated the extent to which the goals and target outcomes documented in the case management plan of care have been achieved

- Demonstrated efficacy, efficiency, quality, safety, and cost-effectiveness of the professional case manager's interventions in achieving the goals documented in the case management plan of care and agreed upon with the client and/or client's family caregiver

- Measured and reported impact of the case management plan of care

- Applied evidence-based adherence guidelines, standardized tools, and proven care processes. These can be used to measure the client's preference for, and understanding of:

    - The proposed case management plan of care and needed resources

    - Motivation to change and demonstrate healthy lifestyle behavior

    - Importance of availability of engaged client, family or family caregiver

- Applied evidence-based guidelines relevant to the care of specific client populations

- Evaluated client and/or client's family or family caregiver experience with case management services

- Used national performance measures for transitional care and care coordination such as those endorsed by the regulatory, accreditation, and certification agencies, and health-related professional associations to ultimately enhance quality, efficiency, and optimal client experience

G. Standard: Closure of Professional Case Management Services

The professional case manager should appropriately complete closure of professional case management services based upon established case closure guidelines. The extent of applying these guidelines may differ in various case management practice and/or care settings.

How demonstrated:

- Achieved care goals and target outcomes, including those self-identified by the client and/or client's family or family caregiver

- Identified reasons for and appropriateness of closure of case management services, such as:
  - Reaching maximum benefit from case management services
  - Change of health care setting which warrants the transition of the client's care to another health care provider(s) and/or setting
  - The employer or purchaser of professional case management services requests the closure of case management
  - Services no longer meet program or benefit eligibility requirements
  - Client refuses further case management services
  - Determination by the professional case manager that he/she is no longer able to provide appropriate case management services because of situations such as a client's ongoing disengagement in self-management and unresolved nonadherence to the case management plan of care
  - Death of the client
  - There is a conflict of interest
  - When a dual relationship raises ethical concerns
- Evidence of agreement for closure of case management services by the client, family or family caregiver, payer, professional case manager, and/or other appropriate parties
- Evidence that when a barrier to closure of professional case management services arises, the case manager has discussed the situation with the appropriate stakeholders and has reached agreement on a plan to resolve the barrier
- Documented reasonable notice for closure of professional case management services and actual closure that is based upon the facts and circumstances of each individual client's case, and care outcomes supporting case closure; evidence should show verbal and/or written notice of case closure to the client and other directly involved health care professionals and support service providers

- Evidence of client education about service and/or funding resources provided by the professional case manager to address any further needs of the client upon case closure

- Completed transition of care handover to health care providers at the next level of care, where appropriate, with permission from client, and inclusive of communication of relevant client information and continuity of the case management plan of care to optimize client care outcomes

H. Standard: Facilitation, Coordination, and Collaboration

The professional case manager should facilitate coordination, communication, and collaboration with the client, client's family or family caregiver, involved members of the interprofessional health care team, and other stakeholders, in order to achieve target goals and maximize positive client care outcomes.

How demonstrated:

- Recognition of the professional case manager's role and practice setting in relation to those of other providers and organizations involved in the provision of care and case management services to the client

- Developing and sustaining proactive client-centered relationships through open communication with the client, client's family or family caregiver, and other relevant stakeholders, to maximize outcomes and enhance client's safety and optimal care experience

- Evidence of facilitation, coordination, and collaboration to support the transitions of care, including:

  - Transfers to the most appropriate health care provider or care setting are coordinated in a timely and complete manner

  - Documentation reflects the collaborative and transparent communication between the professional case manager and other health care team members, especially during each transition to another level of care within or outside of the client's current setting

- ▪ Use of the case management plan of care, target goals, and client's needs and preferences to guide the facilitation and coordination of services and collaboration among members of the interprofessional health care team, client and client's family or family caregiver is evident

- Adherence to client privacy and confidentiality mandates during all aspects of facilitation, coordination, communication, and collaboration within and outside the client's care setting

- Use of special techniques and strategies such as motivational interviewing, mediation, and negotiation, to facilitate transparent communication and building of effective relationships

- Coordination and implementation of the use of problem-solving skills and techniques to reconcile potentially differing points of view

- Evidence of collaboration that optimizes client outcomes; this may include working with community, local, and state resources, primary care providers, members of the interprofessional health care team, the payer, and other relevant stakeholders

- Evidence of collaborative efforts to maximize adherence to regulatory and accreditation standards within the professional case manager's practice and employment setting

I. Standard: Qualifications for Professional Case Managers

The professional case manager should maintain competence in her/his area(s) of practice by having one of the following:

- Current, active, and unrestricted licensure or certification in a health or human services discipline that allows the professional to conduct an assessment independently as permitted within the scope of practice of the discipline

- In the case of an individual who practices in a state that does not require licensure or certification, the individual must have a baccalaureate or graduate degree in social work or another health or human services field that promotes the physical, psychosocial, and/or vocational well-being of the persons being served. The degree must be from an institution that is fully accredited by a nationally recognized educational accreditation organization

- The individual must have completed a supervised field experience in case management, health, or behavioral health as part of the degree requirements.

How demonstrated:

- Possession of the education, experience, and expertise required for the professional case manager's area(s) of practice
- Compliance with national, state, and/or local laws and regulations that apply to the jurisdiction(s) and discipline(s) in which the professional case manager practices
- Maintenance of competence through participation in relevant and ongoing continuing education, certification, academic study, and internship programs
- Practicing within the professional case manager's area(s) of expertise, making timely and appropriate referrals to, and seeking consultation with, others when needed

Supervision

The professional case manager acts in a supervisory and/or leadership role of other personnel who are unable to function independently due to limitations of license and/or education.

Due to the variation in academic degrees and other educational requirements, it is recommended that individuals interested in pursuing a professional case management career seek guidance as to the appropriate educational preparation and academic degree necessary to practice case management. These interested individuals may seek the Case Management Society of America, American Nurses Association, or Commission for Case Manager Certification, or other relevant professional organizations for further advice and guidance.

NOTE: *Social workers who are prepared at the master's in social work (MSW) degree level and educated under a program that would preclude them from sitting for licensure (where required) or practice at the clinical level should consult with their state licensing board to determine if additional educational and/or practicum hours are required.*

J. Standard: Legal

The professional case manager shall adhere to all applicable federal, state, and local laws and regulations that have full force and effect of law, governing all aspects of case management practice including, but not limited to, client privacy and confidentiality rights. It is the responsibility of the professional case manager to work within the scope of his/her license and/or underlying profession.

NOTE: *In the event that the professional case manager's employer policies or those of other entities are in conflict with applicable legal requirements, the case manager should understand that the law prevails. In these situations, case managers should seek clarification of questions or concerns from an appropriate and reliable expert resource, such as a legal counsel, compliance officer, or an appropriate governmental agency.*

1. Standard: Confidentiality and Client Privacy

The professional case manager should adhere to federal, state, and local laws, as well as policies and procedures, governing client privacy and confidentiality, and should act in a manner consistent with the client's best interest in all aspects of communication and record-keeping whether through traditional paper records and/or electronic health records (EHR).

NOTE: *Federal law preempts (supersedes) state and local law and provides a minimum mandatory national standard; states may enlarge client rights, but not reduce them. For those who work exclusively on federal enclaves or on tribal lands, any issues of concern should be directed to the licensing authority and/or federal law.*

How demonstrated:

- Demonstration of up-to-date knowledge of, and adherence to, applicable laws and regulations concerning confidentiality, privacy, and protection of the client's medical information
- Evidence of a good faith effort to obtain the client's written acknowledgment that she/he has received notice of privacy rights and practices

2. Standard: Consent for Professional Case Management Services

The professional case manager should obtain appropriate and informed consent before the implementation of case management services.

How demonstrated:

- Evidence that the client and/or client's family or family caregiver have been thoroughly informed with regard to:
    - Proposed case management process and services relating to the client's health condition(s) and needs
    - Possible benefits and costs of such services
    - Alternatives to proposed services
    - Potential risks and consequences of proposed services and alternatives
    - Client's right to refuse the proposed case management services and awareness of potential risks and consequences of such refusal
- Evidence that the information was communicated in a client-sensitive manner, which is intended to permit the client to make voluntary and informed choices
- Documented informed consent where client consent is a prerequisite to the provision of case management services

K. Standard: Ethics

The professional case manager should behave and practice ethically, and adhere to the tenets of the code of ethics that underlie his/her professional credentials (e.g., nursing, social work, and rehabilitation counseling).

How demonstrated:

- Awareness of the five basic ethical principles and how they are applied. These are:
    - Beneficence (to do good)
    - Nonmaleficence (to do no harm)
    - Autonomy (to respect individuals' rights to make their own decisions),

- Justice (to treat others fairly)
- Fidelity (to follow-through and to keep promises)
- Recognition that:
  - A primary obligation is to the clients cared for
  - A secondary obligation is engagement in and maintenance of respectful relationships with coworkers, employers, and other professionals
  - Laws, rules, policies, insurance benefits, and regulations are sometimes in conflict with ethical principles. In such situations, the professional case manager is bound to address the conflicts to the best of her/his abilities and/or seek appropriate consultation
  - All clients are unique individuals and the professional case manager engages them without regard to gender identity, race or ethnicity, religious practice, other cultural preferences, or socioeconomic status
- Maintaining policies that are universally respectful of the integrity and worth of each person

L. Standard: Advocacy

The professional case manager should advocate for the client, client's family or family caregiver, at the service delivery, benefits administration, and policy-making levels. The case manager is uniquely positioned as an expert in care coordination and advocacy for health policy change to improve access to quality, safe, and cost-effective services.

How demonstrated:

- Documentation demonstrating:
  - Promotion of the client's self-determination, informed and shared decision-making, autonomy, growth, and self-advocacy
  - Education of other health care and service providers in recognizing and respecting the needs, strengths, and goals of the client

- Facilitation of client access to necessary and appropriate services while educating the client and family or family caregiver about resource availability within practice settings

- Recognition, prevention, and elimination of disparities in accessing high-quality care and experiencing optimal client health care outcomes, as related to: race, ethnicity, national origin, and migration background; sex and marital status; age, religion, and political belief; physical, mental, or cognitive disability; gender identity or gender expression; or other cultural factors

- Advocacy for expansion or establishment of services and for client-centered changes in organizational and governmental policy

  - Ensuring a culture of safety by engagement in quality improvement initiatives in the workplace

  - Encouraging the establishment of client, family and/or family caregiver advisory councils to improve client-centered care standards within the organization

  - Joining relevant professional organizations in call to action campaigns, whenever possible, to improve the quality of care and reduce health disparities

- Recognition that client advocacy can sometimes conflict with a need to balance cost constraints and limited resources. Documentation indicates that the professional case manager has weighed decisions with the intent to uphold client advocacy, whenever possible.

M. Standard: Cultural Competence

The professional case manager should maintain awareness of and be responsive to cultural and linguistic diversity of the demographics of her/his work setting and to the specific client and/or caregiver needs.
How demonstrated:

- Evidence of communicating in an effective, respectful, and sensitive manner, and in accordance with the client's cultural and linguistic context

- Assessments, goal-setting, and development of a case management plan of care to accommodate each client's cultural and linguistic needs and preference of services

- Identified appropriate resources to enhance the client's access to care and improve health care outcomes; these may include the use of interpreters and health educational materials that apply language and format demonstrative of understanding of the client's cultural and linguistic communication patterns, including, but not limited to, speech volume, context, tone, kinetics, space, and other similar verbal/nonverbal communication patterns

- Pursuit of professional education to maintain and advance one's level of cultural competence and effectiveness while working with diverse client populations

N. Standard: Resource Management and Stewardship

The professional case manager should integrate factors related to quality, safety, access, and cost-effectiveness in assessing, planning, implementing, monitoring, and evaluating health resources for client care.

How demonstrated:

- Documented evaluation of safety, effectiveness, cost, and target outcomes when designing a case management plan of care to promote the ongoing care needs of the client

- Evidence of follow-through on the objectives of the case management plan of care which are based on the ongoing care needs of the client and the competency, knowledge, and skills of the professional case manager

- Application of evidence-based guidelines and practice recommendations, when appropriate, in recommending resource allocation and utilization options

- Evidence of linking the client and family or family caregiver with cultural and linguistically appropriate resources to meet the needs and goals identified in the case management plan of care

- Documented communication with the client and family or family caregiver about the length of time for availability of a necessary resource, potential and actual financial responsibility associated with a resource, and the range of outcomes associated with resource utilization

- Documented communication with the client and other interprofessional health care team members, especially during care transitions or when there is a significant change in the client's situation
- Evidence of promoting the most effective and efficient use of health care services and financial resources
- Documentation that reflects that the intensity of case management services rendered corresponds with the needs of the client

O. Standard: Professional Responsibilities and Scholarship

The professional case manager should engage in scholarly activities and maintain familiarity with current knowledge, competencies, case management–related research, and evidence-supported care innovations. The professional case manager should also identify best practices in case management and health care and service delivery, and apply such in transforming practice, as appropriate.

How demonstrated:

- Incorporation of current and relevant research findings into one's practice, including policies, procedures, care protocols or guidelines, and workflow processes, and as applicable to the care setting
- Efficient retrieval and appraisal of research evidence that is pertinent to one's practice and client population served
- Proficiency in the application of research-related and evidence-based practice tools and terminologies
- Ability to distinguish peer-reviewed material (e.g., research results, publications) and apply preference to such work in practice, as available and appropriate;
- Accountability and responsibility for own professional development and advancement

- Participation in ongoing training and/or educational opportunities (e.g., conferences, webinars, academic programs) to maintain and expand one's skills, knowledge, and competencies

- Participation in research activities that support quantification and definition of valid and reliable outcomes, especially those that demonstrate the value of case management services and their impact on the individual client and population health

- Identification and evaluation of best practices and innovative case management interventions

- Leveraging opportunities in the employment setting to conduct innovative performance improvement projects and formally report on their results

- Dissemination, through publication and/or presentation at conferences, of practice innovations, research findings, evidence-based practices, and quality or process performance improvement efforts

- Membership in professional case management–related associations and involvement in local, regional, or national committees and task forces

- Mentoring and coaching of less experienced case managers, other interprofessional health care team members, and providers

Interdisciplinary Case Management Team

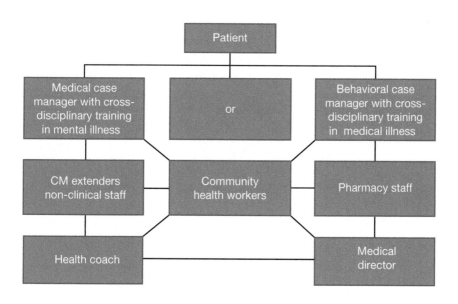

Triggers for Integrated Case Management Intervention

Sources

Data
Screenings, assessment, and self-reporting

Data

- Predictive modeling
  - Determines future risk based on past utilization
  - Diagnoses
  - Population health categorization
  - Identification of missing preventative or needed services
- Utilization
  - Inpatient admissions
  - Length of stay
  - Emergency department visits
  - Medication adherence
    - Medications filled as ordered
  - Diagnoses
    - Medical conditions
    - Mental illness
    - Behavioral conditions

- Reports
    - State reporting of special needs populations
        - Long-term support services recipients
        - Individuals diagnosed with intellectual/developmental disabilities
        - Children in foster care
        - Waiver recipients
        - Other special needs populations

Screenings, Assessments, and Self-Reporting

- Self-assessment
- Comprehensive assessment conducted by professional case manager
- Family/caregiver referral
- Physician referral
- Other provider or community referral

Adult Integrated Case Management Complexity Grid

ICM-CAG

Date:	HEALTH RISKS AND HEALTH NEEDS					
Name:	HISTORICAL		CURRENT STATE		VULNERABILITY	
Total Score =	Complexity Item	Score	Complexity Item	Score	Complexity Item	Score
Biological Domain	Chronic Illness		Symptom Severity/ Impairment		Complications and Life Threat	
	Diagnostic Difficulty		Adherence Ability			
Psychological Domain	Barriers to Coping		Resistance to Treatment		Mental Health Threat	
	Mental Health History		Mental Health Symptoms			
Social Domain	Job and Leisure		Residential Stability		Social Vulnerability	
	Relationships		Social Support			

(continued)

Date:	HEALTH RISKS AND HEALTH NEEDS				
Name:	HISTORICAL		CURRENT STATE		VULNERABILITY
Health System Domain	Access to Care		Getting Needed Services		Health System Deterrents
	Treatment Experience		Provider Collaboration		
Comments					
(Enter pertinent information about the reason for the score of each complexity item *here* (e.g., poor patient adherence, death in family with stress to patient, non-evidence-based treatment of *migraine*)					
Scoring System Green: 0 = no need to act Yellow: 1 = mild risk and need for monitoring or prevention Orange: 2 = moderate risk and need for action or development of intervention plan Red: 3 = severe risk and need for immediate action or immediate intervention plan					

Note: Permission for re-use must be obtained from the authors by contacting ICM@cmsa.org.

Adult Integrated Case Management Complexity Grid Elements and Rating Scales

BIOLOGICAL DOMAIN ITEMS		PSYCHOLOGICAL DOMAIN ITEMS	
Chronic Illness	Physical illness chronicity	Barriers to Coping	Problems handling stress and/or problem solving
Diagnostic Difficulty	Difficulty getting a condition diagnosed; multiple providers consulted; multiple diagnostic tests completed	Mental Health History	Prior mental condition difficulties
Symptom Severity	Physical illness symptom severity and impairment; does the severity of symptoms result in a disability, i.e., unable to care for self, unable to perform ADL or IADL, unable to work or go to school	Resistance to Treatment	Resistance to treatment/ nonadherence; doesn't believe the treatment is right for him/ her; not following a physician's treatment plan due to poor health literacy/doesn't understand the goal of treatment; or a behavioral condition has interfered, i.e., depression, anxiety, poorly managed SMI
Adherence Ability	Current difficulties in the ability to follow a physician's treatment plan	Mental Health Symptoms	Current mental condition symptom severity
Complications and Life Threat	Risk of physical complications and life threat if case management is stopped	Mental Health Threat	Risk of persistent personal barriers or poor mental condition care if case management is stopped

(*continued*)

SOCIAL DOMAIN ITEMS		HEALTH SYSTEM DOMAIN ITEMS	
Job and Leisure	Personal productivity and leisure activities; employed in the last 6 months; function as a caregiver, full-time parent, and/or homemaker; attend school; have leisure activities like hobbies, participation in social groups, regular outings with friends and family	Access to Care	Access to care and services as they relate to insurance coverage, financial responsibility, language, culture, geography; use of the ED instead of establishing a relationship with a physician(s) or another provider(s)
Relationships	Healthy relationships; relationship difficulties; ability to maintain relationships with spouse, family, neighbors, friends, coworkers; presence of dysfunctional relationships; physical altercations with others	Treatment Experience	Experiences with doctors, hospitals, or health system
Residential Stability	Residential stability or suitability; ability to meet financial obligations (rent, mortgage, utilities); access to food, clothing, etc.; housing is safe	Getting Needed Services	Logistical ability to get needed care: getting appointments, transportation to/from appointments; use of the ED instead of seeing outpatient providers; seeing providers who accept cultural practices and/or speak the patient's primary language
Social Support	Availability of social support: have help available when needed or wanted from family, friends, coworkers, other social contacts (e.g., church members) or community supports (e.g., peer support, community health worker)	Provider Collaboration	Communication among providers to ensure coordinated care
Social Vulnerability	Risk of work, loss of income, home, and relational support needs if case management is stopped	Health System Deterrents	Risk of continued poor access to and/or coordination of services if case management is stopped

ADL, activities of daily living; ED, emergency department; IADL, instrumental activities of daily living; SMI, serious mental illness.

Timeframes

- History
- Current status
- Future risk

Biological Domain

Chronic Illness

0 = Less than 3 months of physical dysfunction and/or an acute condition
- No action required

1 = More than 3 months of physical dysfunction, or intermittent dysfunction for the last 3 months (i.e., pain, loss of appetite)
- Review with the patient his or her understanding of why this dysfunction has occurred; the cause of the dysfunction
- Will need to observe over time to see if the dysfunction becomes a chronic condition
- Ensure that patient is following up with the primary care or specialty provider

2 = Presence of a chronic disease/illness
- Review with the patient his or her understanding of the condition and treatment
- Assist the patient in simplifying management if it appears needed
- Ensure the patient is keeping medical appointments
- Evaluate control of the condition by reviewing any symptoms and what metrics are regularly completed (e.g., for patients with diabetes, when was the last HgA1c completed and the results; for a patient with hypertension, how often is blood pressure checked and what was the most recent reading)

3 = More than one chronic disease/illness
- Complete activities for Risk Level 2
- Customize any actions related to the results of the assessment, e.g., the patient has not had an HgA1c in over a year—important

to schedule as soon as possible; a member with heart disease who states he or she has intermittent chest pain—schedule an appointment with the provider as soon as possible, or refer to the emergency department (ED) if having acute symptoms

- Evaluate the number of providers involved in the patient's care and report findings to the treating providers ensuring all are aware

Diagnostic Difficulty

0 = No difficulty with the diagnosis of a condition; diagnosis was made easily, e.g., blood pressure has been elevated for 3 months

- No action needed

1 = A diagnosis was arrived at relatively quickly, e.g., patient exhibiting flu-like symptoms and a localized rash—blood test revealed ehrlichiosis from a tick bite

- Observe for any changes in the patient's clinical status

2 = Diagnosis made but only after considerable diagnostic work-up, e.g., patient diagnosed with multiple sclerosis (MS) but only after blood work, MRI, and spinal tap

- Review with the patient his or her understanding of the condition(s), prescribed treatment, what improvements are expected, and over what time frame

- Assess how the patient managed the diagnostic period

- Discuss what we can do to support the patient to experience a positive outcome

- If the patient is having difficulty with the diagnosis, ask if he or she has discussed this with the physician(s) and would the patient like for us as the case manager to communicate his or her concerns

3 = After significant diagnostic work-up, no firm diagnosis has been made

- Complete all actions under Risk Level 2 immediately

- Customize any interventions based on what we learn

- Ask the patient what concerns his or her the most about not reaching a diagnosis

- Offer to communicate these concerns to all involved providers

Symptom Severity and Impairment

0 = No physical symptoms or symptoms are resolved by treatment, e.g., migraine headaches are controlled by regularly scheduled Botox injections

- No action required other than to observe efficacy of current treatment

1 = Mild symptoms, but do not interfere with daily function, e.g., arthritic pain in hands but still able to knit and crochet, able to work in the garden

- Observe for worsening symptoms

2 = Moderate symptoms that interfere with daily functions, e.g., chronic back pain that requires rest and analgesics; may miss 1 to 3 days of work

- Ensure primary care and other involved providers are aware of symptoms
- Ensure patient is following up with providers as required
- Be aware of any follow-up testing that may be ordered for worsening symptoms
- Make sure patient understands condition, what to report to providers, when to seek immediate care
- If assistive interventions are required, assist in facilitation and coordination

3 = Severe symptoms that result in an inability to perform many daily functions, e.g., patient with chronic obstructive pulmonary disease (COPD) unable to climb the stairs to the second floor of his or her home, vacuum the floors, or walk one block to the market; a patient with MS is chair bound and requires assistance to bathe and use the toilet

- Complete actions from Risk Levels 1 and 2 immediately
- Update the patient's providers with any concerns or risks
- Customize other actions based on what was learned from the assessment
- Assess what current interventions help the patient most; what is working
- Assess what is not working; where challenges lie
- Evaluate the presence of social support that can aid with those activities too difficult for the patient to perform or complete

- Facilitate and coordinate, with collaboration from the treating physician, services that might result in comfort or improvement: rehabilitation, home care

Adherence Ability

0 = Ability to follow a treatment plan; the treatment plan is uncomplicated

1 = The treatment plan is slightly complicated but the client can follow

2 = The treatment plan is slightly complicated but the client has difficulty following. The client needs support and motivation to adhere

3 = The client is unable to follow the prescribed treatment plan due to physical symptoms or has behavioral conditions that interfere with the ability to adhere

Vulnerability and Life Threat

0 = Little to no risk of worsening physical symptoms and/or limitations in activities of daily living

- No action required

1 = Mild risk of worsening physical symptoms and/or limitations in activities of daily living

- Encourage adherence to treatment and observe for any barriers that may appear
- Work with patient to remove barriers

2 = Moderate risk of worsening physical symptoms and/or substantial limitations in activities of daily living

- Work with the patient to address any causes for nonadherence
- If behavioral conditions are a cause, work to coordinate needed behavioral services
- Ensure patient and provider are communicating and each understands each other's goals and concerns.
- Monitor appropriate clinical tests and utilization, e.g., blood sugar, blood pressure, blood chemistries, scans, admissions, ED visits
- Case management intervention may be intermittent or long term

3 = Severe risk of physical complications associated with permanent loss of function and/or risk of death

- Perform actions under Risk Level 2
- Customize actions based on assessment
- Perform frequent reassessment of physical symptoms and response to prescribed treatment
- Case management intervention will need to continue until risks are reduced or mitigated
- If appropriate, coordinate long-term, palliative, or hospice care

Psychological Domain

Barriers to Coping

0 = The ability to manage stress, life situations, and health concerns by seeking support or participating in activities that result in relaxation and satisfaction, e.g., seeking medical advice, hobbies, social activities

- No action required

1 = Limited coping skills such as a need for control, denial of illness, irritability

- Help the patient identify stressors and supports for stressful situations
- Encourage counseling to gain insight into positive coping strategies

2 = Impaired coping skills such as chronic complaining, substance use (self-medication) but without serious impact on medical conditions, mental health, or social situation

- Encourage counseling to gain insight into positive coping strategies that may include specific stress-reduction techniques or conflict resolution training
- Recommend Employee Assistance Program (EAP) for any work-related stressors
- If living arrangements, work location, or social activities seem too stressful, discuss with patient strategies to change to reduce stressors
- Screen for alcohol abuse if needed

- Consider reaching out to the patient's primary care physician (PCP) if substance/alcohol abuse is of concern or if the patient may benefit from a mental health professional referral

3 = Poor or absent coping skills manifested by destructive behavior like substance abuse/dependence, psychiatric illness, self-mutilation, suicide attempts, failed/failing social relationships

- Perform actions under Risk Level 2
- Customize actions based on what was learned in the assessment
- Assist in the development of a crisis intervention plan that may include the patient's support system and providers
- Collaborate with providers for a mental health referral for assessment and treatment recommendations
- Support and encourage mental health treatment with the patient
- Collaborate with the PCP for a referral to substance/alcohol abuse treatment
- Support and encourage participation in substance/alcohol abuse treatment

Mental Health History

0 = No history of mental health problems or conditions

- No action required

1 = Mental health problems or conditions, but resolved or without clear effects on daily function

- Encourage regular primary care screenings for mental conditions with intervention, if appropriate
- Check for access to support from mental health professionals

2 = Mental health conditions that have clear effects on daily function, the need for therapy, medication, day treatment, or a partial inpatient program

- Ensure the patient's understanding of potential for recurrence of mental health conditions by using lay language
- Understand the potential for medical and physical condition interactions, if indicated
- Facilitate and coordinate visits and regular follow-up with a psychiatrist and/or mental health team (psychologists, social

workers, nurses, substance use disorder and other counselors) provide support when conditions destabilize

- Facilitate, coordinate, and support follow-up with the PCP
- Refer to a medical home, if available, to ensure all needed services are provided in one setting
- Monitor patient symptoms over time (e.g., PHQ-9, GAD-7)
- Assist with communication among physical and mental health–treating clinicians

3 = Psychiatric admissions and/or persistent effects on daily function due to mental illness

- Perform actions under Risk Level 2
- Include customized actions based on interview
- Facilitate communication between the mental health team for mental conditions and with the PCPs who care for concurrent physical illness
- Collaborate with providers to develop transition plans that will prevent readmissions
- Support, encourage, and assist the patient to make and keep appointments with providers, especially mental health providers
- Facilitate and coordinate any outpatient services ordered by the treating physician to help stabilize the patient's mental illness(es)
- Facilitate and coordinate appropriate social supports for the patient to prevent symptom exacerbation and readmission

Resistance to Treatment

0 = Interested in receiving treatment and willing to cooperate actively

- No action required

1 = Some ambivalence or hesitation, though willing to cooperate with prescribed treatment

- Educate patient/family about illnesses
- Initiate discussions with patient about willingness to recognize conditions and prescribed treatments using motivational interviewing and problem-solving techniques to facilitate change

- Explore other barriers to treatment adherence
- Inform providers of adherence problems and work with them to consider alternative interventions, if needed

2 = Considerable resistance and nonadherence; hostility or indifference toward health care professionals, diagnosed conditions, and/or treatments

- Perform actions under Risk Level 1
- Actively explore and attempt to reverse other sources of resistance (e.g., family member's negativism, religious objections, cultural influences, relationships with treating physician)

3 = Active resistance to important medical care

- Perform actions under Risk Levels 1 and 2
- Include customized actions based on interview
- Collaborate with treating clinicians in considering and instituting alternative interventions
- If needed, work with case management medical director to find second opinion practitioners
- If significant resistance exists and is pervasive, consider discontinuation of case management

Mental Health Symptoms

0 = No mental health symptoms

- No action needed

1 = Mild mental health symptoms, such as problems with concentration or feeling tense or nervous but do not interfere with current functioning

- Ensure the patient is receiving primary care treatment with access to support from mental health professionals
- Facilitate communication between all treating providers

2 = Moderate mental health symptoms, such as anxiety, depression, or mild cognitive impairment that interfere with current functioning

- Perform actions under Risk Level 1
- Ensure that acute, maintenance, and continuation of treatment is being provided by PCPs with mental health support
- Facilitate primary maintenance and continuation treatment provided by PCP in a medical home if possible, with

mental health specialist assistance—that is, a psychiatrist and mental health team (psychologists, social workers, nurses, substance abuse counselors, et al.)—when condition destabilizes, becomes complicated, or demonstrates treatment resistance

- Evaluate and assess symptoms and document using the PHQ-9, GAD-7, and patient report; report concerns to providers
- Develop a crisis plan with the patient and with provider input

3 = Severe psychiatric symptoms and/or behavioral disturbances, such as violence, self-inflicted harm, delirium, criminal behavior, psychosis, or mania

- Perform actions under Risk Levels 1 and 2
- Include customized actions based on interview
- Support active and aggressive treatment for mental conditions by a mental health team working in close collaboration with PCPs, who care for concurrent physical illness
- When possible, encourage geographically colocated physical and mental health personnel to facilitate ease of coordinating treatment; e.g., medical home or practices in the same vicinity
- Evaluate and assess symptoms and document using the PHQ-9, GAD-7, and patient report; report any concerns immediately to providers

Mental Health Risk and Vulnerability

0 = No evidence of risk

1 = Mild risk of worsening mental health/behavioral symptoms

- Facilitate and coordinate access to appropriate mental health supports and services
- Support and encourage follow-up care with providers and perform intermittent mental health assessments, to monitor symptoms, i.e., PHQ-9, GAD-7
- Encourage and support coping and stress reduction activates; can be formal or informal

2 = Moderate risk of worsening mental health symptoms
- Perform actions under Risk Level 1
- Assist the patient in knowing where and from whom to get assistance: PCP, psychiatrist, counselor, et al.
- Assess symptoms related to depression and anxiety by using tools such as PHQ-9, GAD-7
- Facilitate communication between medical and behavioral providers as necessary; facilitate access to an integrated medical home if possible
- Promote and encourage adherence to prescribed treatment
- Involve caregivers of the patient if agreeable and consent received, in all activities

3 = Severe and persistent risk of psychiatric disorder with frequent health service use
- Perform actions under Risk Levels 1 and 2
- Include interventions that are specific to the patient's prescribed treatment: medication, therapy, or other more aggressive interventions
- Work with the patient's clinicians to understand the clinical goals and assist the patient with understanding and with removal of barriers to achieve goals
- Patient may need long-term case management involvement

Social Domain

Job and Leisure

0 = Patient has a "job" which includes employment, furthering education, stay-at-home parent or homemaker, leisure activates that include clubs, hobbies, travel, sports
- No action required.

1 = Patient has a job (as just described) but without leisure activities
- Discuss with the patient past experiences with leisure activity

2 = Patient has leisure activates but does not have a job now or for the last 6 months
- Discuss with member his/her ability to work, willingness to work, or go to school

- Make referrals to appropriate resources; social security for disability, social services for educational and vocational resources
- If unable to return to work, provide information on how to access public assistance programs
- Follow up timely to ensure the patient has been able to access any needed resources and assist as necessary
- Encourage any interest in leisure activities

3 = No job for more than 6 months and without leisure activities
- Perform activities under Risk Levels 1 and 2
- Explore the impact of not having a job and income in ability to access health services
- Access to public assistance may be more of an urgency; look for community resources that could assist in the interim

Relationships

0 = No social disruptions; no dysfunctional relationships

1 = Mild social disruptions or interpersonal problems; you may argue with family or friends but usually resolve differences with time
- If possible, observe the patient's interactions with family or providers

2 = Moderate social dysfunction, social relationships are tenuous, no strong friendships or family ties, would rather be alone
- Encourage member to include family or other supporting acquaintances to be involved in care
- Assess if social issues have any impact on the patient's health, e.g., has no one to call when sick
- Assess if the patient is open to work with a counselor to improve social skills
- Explore with patient if there are social activities in which he/ she might be willing to participate

3 = Severe social dysfunction, social isolation, unable to "get along" with family, friends, coworkers, neighbors; argumentative, hostile
- Complete actions from Risk Levels 1 and 2
- Facilitate behavioral health assessment due to disruptive and/or destructive behaviors

Residential Stability

0 = Stable housing, stable living arrangements, able to live independently

- No action required

1 = Stable housing with support of others, e.g., family available to assist, receiving home care or home and community-based services, or living in an institutional setting like assisted living, group home, or long-term care facility

- Facilitate and coordinate additional support where and when needed; this may require looking for community supports when services are not reimbursed, e.g., church volunteers, extended family, friends or coworkers willing to provide support
- Frequent assessments for potential changes in the patient's needs

2 = Unstable housing, e.g., no support at home or living in a shelter; inability to meet financial obligations related to housing; there is a need to change the current housing situation

- Consult with social services or community housing resources to explore housing options
- Consult with social services or community resources to assist with meeting financial obligations; explore with member the willingness to include family and friends in proving more support
- Be timely with follow-up on availability and coordination of needed resources

3 = No current satisfactory or safe housing, e.g., homeless, transient housing (couch surfing), or dangerous environment; an immediate change is required

- Immediately connect the patient with safe housing (e.g., emergency shelter or shelter with trusted individual)
- Follow up with options as soon as the patient is safe for safe housing: consult with social services and/or community housing resources
- Follow-up on coordination of safe housing is a prioritized action
- If appropriate, contact housing authority for needed repairs or mitigation of other unsafe living situations unrelated to violence (e.g., vermin or insect infestations, unsafe structures)

Social Support

0 = Assistance is readily available from family, friends, coworkers, acquaintances (e.g., church or club members), always

- No action required

1 = Assistance is generally available from family, friends, coworkers, or acquaintances; assistance may be sporadic and not always available when needed

- Assess what assistance is needed

- Discuss with patient and social supports, who can assist and when

- Develop contingency plan for assistance when no one is available: e.g., transportation to appointments, what so do in an emergency.

2 = Limited assistance from family, friends, coworkers, acquaintances (e.g., family does not live close, patient has a limited social circle)

- Discuss with patient and social supports, who can assist and when

- Develop contingency plan for assistance when no one is available: e.g., transportation to appointments, what so do in an emergency.

- Assess for in-home support by home health agencies or volunteer organizations if appropriate

3 = No assistance is available from family, friends, coworkers, acquaintances at any time

- Assess for the need and availability of in-home supports, e.g., home- and community-based services

- Coordinate needed transportation, access to food

- Discuss with patient and providers the need for transfer to a setting that will provide more safety and support (e.g., assisted living, group home).

Social Vulnerability

0 = No risk present that warrants the need to change the living situation; social supports are present; and the patient can meet financial obligations

- No action required

1 = Some assistance might be needed to ensure social supports are available when needed

- Work with member to determine if current supports will be available in the future
- If in-home supports are needed, determine the length of time needed and availability of the services for that period
- Make sure contingency plan is developed for long term

2 = Risk exists that would result in the patient having little to no social support, will be unable to meet financial obligations, keep medical appointments

- Work with the patient and support system to determine if support will continue regardless of how limited
- Explore availability of community and social resources to assist with financial obligations, access to food: Is there a limit to what can be accessed?
- Review benefits/reimbursement to ensure any coordinated services can be extended long term
- If unable to extend in-home services, community resources, and social support, explore placement options

3 = Immediate, and into the next few months, need for placement of supports, assistance with meeting financial obligations, emergency planning, and/or placement in a safe environment

- All actions under Risk Level 2 need to be completed as soon as possible
- Expedite placement to a safe environment if home-based options are not feasible

Health System Domain

Access to Care

0 = Adequate access to care: no issues with insurance, reasonable premiums, coinsurance, co-pays; providers are available near the patient, the patient can make and keep appointments

- No action required

1 = Some difficulty accessing care; long travel to providers; limited access to specialists like psychiatrists; long waits to get appointments; high pharmacy co-pays; providers who meet preferred cultural practice or language or not available

- Assist the patient in researching providers who meet their preferences for culture or language
- Assist patients in making appointments
- Discuss medications with high co-pays with pharmacy staff or medical director to see if peer-to-peer could result in more affordable medication

2 = Difficulty accessing care due to geography, language, culture, insurance coverage, or premiums (see detail in #1)

- All activities in #1 should be completed but with the case manager taking a more active role in helping the patient locate the preferred providers
- Speak with provider offices to facilitate expedited appointments or coordinate multiple appointments in 1 day so that travel is reduced
- Assist with filling gaps in care (e.g., lack of counselors: facilitate telephone, Skype, or other telecommunications for access to counseling services)
- If insurance costs are too high, explore what other options may be available to the patient

3 = No adequate access to care due to geography, language, culture, insurance coverage or premiums (see details in #1)

- Expedite activities in #2
- Contact social services to see if the patient might qualify for access to specialty clinics

Treatment Experience

0 = No problems with health care providers

- No action required

1 = Negative experiences with health care providers

- Ask the patient to describe the experiences
- Ask the patient if he or she could follow recommended treatment plans

- Ask the patient to describe what kind of provider he or she would like to see
- Help the patient better prepare for provider visits by helping the patient develop questions to ask the provider; recommend the patient write down the questions to take to appointments

2 = Multiple providers; has changed providers many times due to dissatisfaction or sees multiple providers

- Complete the actions in #1
- Have the patient describe the conflicts and then assist the patient in resolving conflicts with practitioners if possible by communicating the patient's concerns to the provider
- Review the recommended treatment plan with the patient, ask if this is a plan he or she can follow; if not, why not; and to facilitate communication of those concerns with the provider
- If conflicts do not seem to be resolved, ask the medical director to speak with the provider
- If the patient is still not happy with provider, help the patient find a new provider

3 = Repeated provider conflicts/ED use

- Complete actions under #2
- Speak with providers to see if a mental health evaluation is warranted
- Offer to coordinate conflict resolution training and strategies for the patients

Provider Collaboration

0 = Patient able to communicate effectively with all practitioners and practitioners communicate with each other; there are no problems with coordination of care

- No action required

1 = Primary care practitioner coordinates all care including mental health services; limited communication if patient has more than one practitioner

- Review with patient if mental health practitioner is needed

- Communicate with PCP that mental health professional services can be coordinated
- Make the patient aware that integrated practices are available: patient-centered medical home (PCMH) or health home
- Facilitate communication between practitioners, provide medication lists, appointment dates, etc.

2 = Lack of communication among providers related to a patient's conditions and ordered treatment

- Implement actions under #1
- Help the patient schedule same-day appointments for different problems. Patient can be instructed to bring summary of each visit to the next
- Communicate with all practitioners that you can facilitate co-ordination of needed care and services
- Suggest accessing care at an integrated clinic (PCMH or health home)

3 = No communication among providers and no responsible party for care coordination

- Implement all actions under #2
- Attend provider visits with the patient if possible
- Speak with treating practitioners on behalf of the patient, with the patient's permission (may need to have written consent)

Health System Deterrents/Vulnerability

0 = No risk or concern that care between medical and behavioral is not coordinated; no issues with insurance or financial

- No action required

1 = Mild risk of health system challenges such as insurance coverage restrictions, geographical access to care, inconsistent or limited communication between providers, or inconsistent coordination of care

- Examine with the patient any insurance coverage restrictions or deterrents like high deductible, or coinsurance, exclusions
- Investigate community resources for services not covered by insurance (e.g., counseling, other mental health services)

- Determine with the patient if they have the resources to maintain insurance coverage
- If there is a threat to maintaining coverage, strategize how to mitigate that threat
- Is it possible for the patient to continue to see providers who are not geographically convenient?
- Continue to facilitate communication between providers

2 = Moderate risk of health system challenges related to insurance coverage restrictions, potential loss of insurance coverage, geographical access to care, poor communication among providers, and poor care coordination

- Complete actions in #1
- Assist with finding resources to continue affordable health insurance coverage if unable to maintain current coverage
- Facilitate care in a medical home to improve communication and care coordination

3 = Severe risk of health system challenges such as no health insurance, limited coverage, providers resistant to communication, and no obvious coordination of care

- Complete actions in Risk Levels 1 and 2 immediately

Pediatric Integrated Case Management Complexity Grid

PIM-CAG

Date:	HEALTH RISKS AND HEALTH NEEDS					
Name:	HISTORICAL		CURRENT STATE		VULNERABILITY	
Total Score =	Complexity Item	Score	Complexity Item	Score	Complexity Item	Score
Biological Domain	Chronic Illness		Symptom Severity/ Impairment		Complications and Life Threat	
	Diagnostic Difficulty		Adherence Ability			
Psychological Domain	Barriers to Coping		Resistance to Treatment		Learning and/ or Mental Health Threat	
	Mental Health History		Mental Health Symptoms			
	Cognitive Development					
	Adverse Developmental Events					

(continued)

Date:	HEALTH RISKS AND HEALTH NEEDS					
Name:	HISTORICAL		CURRENT STATE		VULNERABILITY	
Total Score =	Complexity Item	Score	Complexity Item	Score	Complexity Item	Score
Social Domain	Learning Ability		Residential Stability		Family/School/ Social System Vulnerability	
	Family and Social Relationships		Child/ Adolescent Support System			
	Caregiver/ Parent Health and Function		Caregiver/ Family Support			
			School and Community Participation			
Health System Domain	Access to Care		Getting Needed Services		Health System Deterrents	
	Treatment Experience		Provider Collaboration			

Scoring System
Green: 0 = no vulnerability or need to act
Yellow: 1 = mild vulnerability and need for monitoring or prevention
Orange: 2 = moderate vulnerability and need for action or development of intervention plan
Red: 3 = severe vulnerability and need for immediate action or immediate intervention plan

Note: Permission for re-use must be obtained from the authors by contacting ICM@cmsa.org.

G

Pediatric Integrated Case Management Complexity Grid Elements and Rating Scales

BIOLOGICAL DOMAIN ITEMS		PSYCHOLOGICAL DOMAIN ITEMS	
Chronic Illness	Presence of chronic physical illness	Barriers to Coping	Problems handling stress or engaging in problem solving
		Mental Health History	Prior mental condition
Diagnostic Difficulty	Difficulty getting a condition diagnosed; multiple providers have been consulted; multiple diagnostic tests completed	Cognitive Development	Cognitive level and capabilities
		Adverse Developmental Events	Early adverse physical and mental health events: complications during pregnancy; other adverse event that took place early in childhood resulting in interrupting cognitive or behavioral development; trauma
Symptom Severity/ Impairment	Physical illness symptom severity and impairment; do the physical symptoms result in a disability, e.g., unable to care for self, ADL, IADL; unable to attend school or participate in any school-related activity, e.g., physical education	Resistance to Treatment	Resistance to treatment; nonadherence; encompasses the parent/guardian and/or the child/adolescent: does not believe the treatment is right for him/her; not following a physician's treatment plan due to poor health, poor health literacy, lack of understanding related to the goal of treatment; a behavioral condition has interfered, e.g., depression, anxiety, poorly managed SMI

(continued)

BIOLOGICAL DOMAIN ITEMS		PSYCHOLOGICAL DOMAIN ITEMS	
Adherence Ability	Current difficulties in the ability to follow a physician's treatment plan by the parent/guardian or the child	Mental Health Symptoms	Current mental conditions with symptom severity; presence of mental health symptoms or challenging behaviors
Complications and Life Threat	Risk of physical complications and life threat if case management is stopped	Learning and/or Mental Health Threat	Risk of persistent personal barriers, cognitive deficits, or poor mental condition care if case management is stopped
SOCIAL DOMAIN ITEMS		HEALTH SYSTEM DOMAIN ITEMS	
Learning Ability	History/presence of learning difficulties, ability to participate in learning activities	Access to Care	Access to care and services as they relate to insurance coverage, financial responsibility, language, geography; use of the ED instead of establishing a relationship with a physician or other provider
Family and Social Relationships	Stability in parent/guardian relationships; ability to make friends, socialize with peers		
Caregiver Health and Function	Caregiver/parent physical and mental health condition and function; ability to support the health and well-being of the child/adolescent	Treatment Experience	Experience with doctors, hospitals, or other areas of the health system
Residential Stability	Food and housing situation; safe place to live, free from abuse, neglect; resources are available to support safe living, financial resources for food, utilities, rent, mortgage	Getting Needed Services	Logistical ability to get needed care: getting appointments, use of the ED instead of seeking outpatient care
Child/Adolescent Support System	Child/youth support system; who is available to support the child?		

(continued)

SOCIAL DOMAIN ITEMS		HEALTH SYSTEM DOMAIN ITEMS	
Caregiver/Family Support System	Caregiver/parent support system; who provides social support to family/caregiver?	Provider Collaboration	Communication among providers to ensure coordinated care
School and Community Participation	Attendance, achievement, and behavior at school		
Family/School/Social Vulnerability	Risk for home/school support or supervision needs if case management is stopped	Health System Deterrents	Risk of continued poor access to and/or coordination of services if case management is stopped

ADL, activities of daily living; ED, emergency department; IADL, instrumental activities of daily living; SMI, serious mental illness.

Timeframes

- History
- Current status
- Future risk

When using the Pediatric Integrated Case Management Complexity Grid (PIM-CAG), assessment is conducted in the four domains but with additional risk elements. Those additional elements are detailed here.

Psychological Domain
Cognitive Development

0 = No cognitive impairment
- No action required

1 = Possible developmental delay or immaturity; low IQ
- Assist in establishing level of impairment, including capacity of child to communicate physical needs and symptoms by coordinating referrals for appropriate testing
- Discuss level of impairment and needs with caregivers, educator, and the pediatrician to ensure appropriate placement in school system

- Assess need for remedial educational assistance and home support; facilitate completion of an individual educational plan (IEP) to meet the child's educational needs

- Maintain communication with the school system and medical providers regarding the child's progress with learning

2 = Delayed development; mild or moderate cognitive impairment

- Complete actions under Risk Level 1

- Review performance/adjustment issues with school facility; involve social services if needed if there is a lack of improvement

- Assess and assist with home support for child/youth based on functional capabilities and respite for caregivers/parents related to assimilation of social skills; provide relief for parents/guardians from day-to-day caregiving

- Assess and share child/youth's ability to communicate

3 = Severe and pervasive developmental delays or profound cognitive impairment

- Complete actions under Risk Levels 1 and 2

- Ensure parents/guardian have access to needed resources and supports to deal with severe developmental delays

- In extreme circumstances, placement may be required. Work with providers and parents/guardian to facilitate a such a difficult transition

Adverse Developmental Events

0 = No identified developmental traumas or injuries (e.g., physical or sexual abuse, meningitis, lead exposure, drug abuse, exposure to infection, or other untoward prenatal exposures)

- No action required

1 = Traumatic prior experiences or injuries with no apparent or stated impact on child/youth

- While at the time of assessment there may appear to be no untoward effects of early trauma or exposure, observation is warranted as the child grows and develops

2 = Traumatic prior experiences or injuries with potential relationship to impairment in child/youth

- Facilitate needed testing and evaluation to the extent that the trauma or exposure has affected the child
- Facilitate appropriate interventions to reduce the resulting effects of the trauma or exposure

3 = Traumatic prior experiences with apparent and significant direct relationship to impairment in child/youth

- Complete actions under Risk Level 2
- Urgently coordinate needed services to address the impairments experienced due to trauma and exposures

Social Domain
Learning Ability

0 = Performing well in school with good achievement, attendance, and behavior

- No action required

1 = Performing adequately in school although there are some achievement, attendance, and behavioral problems (e.g., missed classes, pranks)

- Encourage parents/caregivers to become more closely involved with the child's teachers and administrators

2 = Experiencing moderate problems with school achievement, attendance, and/or behavior (e.g., school disciplinary action, few school-related peer relationships, academic probation)

- Recommend parents/guardians closely work with teachers and counselors to determine strategies to improve achievement, attendance, and reduce disruptive behavior
- May need to refer to additional counseling or tutoring resources outside of school

3 = Experiencing severe problems with school achievement, attendance, and/or behavior (e.g., homebound education, school suspension, violence, illegal activities at school, academic failure, school dropout, disruptive peer group activity)

- Urgently assist with facilitation of additional resources and referrals for counseling, tutoring.

Family and Social Relationships

0 = Stable nurturing home, good social, and peer relationships

- No action is required

1 = Mild family problems, minor problems with social and peer relationships (e.g., parent–child conflict, frequent fights, marital discord, lacking close friends)

- Offer to facilitate counseling to address family problems or the child's challenges with making friends

2 = Moderate level of family problems, inability to initiate and maintain social and peer relationships (e.g., parental neglect, difficult separation/ divorce, alcohol abuse, hostile caregiver, difficulties in maintaining same-age peer relationships)

- Collaborate with providers and school to encourage family counseling or counseling for the child's inability to maintain relationships
- Involve social services to assess family dysfunction and risk to child/adolescent's safety

3 = Severe family problems with disruptive social and peer relationships (e.g., significant abuse, hostile child custody battles, addiction issues, parental criminality, complete social isolation, little, or no association with peers)

- Immediately notify social services or appropriate authorities if there is a risk of danger to the welfare of your patient or other family member
- Notify the patient's providers of concerns with social isolation, facilitate referral to appropriate mental health providers

Caregiver/Parent Health and Function

0 = All caregivers healthy

- No action required

1 = Physical and/or mental health issues, including poor coping skills, and/or permanent disability, present in one or more caregiver that do not impact parenting

- Discuss with parent/guardian the challenges and contributors to difficulty coping and what, if any, resources are available to assist with coping
- Assess any needed assistance related to existing disabilities
- Provide resources to the parent/guardian to obtain defined assistance

2 = Physical and/or mental health conditions, including disrupted coping resources, and/or permanent disability, present in one or more caregiver that interfere with parenting

- Complete actions under Risk Level 1
- Assist parent/guardian in making needed appointments for counseling and other mental health services
- Provide information on resources that may assist the parent/guardian with compensation of any physical disability

3 = Physical and/or mental health conditions, including disrupted coping styles, and/or permanent disability, present in one or more caregiver that prevent effective parenting and/or create a dangerous situation for the child/youth

- Immediately contact the patient's providers to advise of a dangerous situation
- Work with social services to ensure the patient has a safe environment even if just temporary
- Reassure the parent/caregiver that you will assist in making sure there is no interruption in the care and services received by the patient

Child/Adolescent Support

0 = Supervision and/or assistance readily available from family/caregiver, friends/peers, teachers, and/or community social networks (e.g., spiritual/religious groups) at all times

- No action required

1 = Supervision and/or assistance generally available from family/caregiver, friends/peers, teachers, and/or community social networks; but possible delays

- Ascertain who, besides parent/guardian, are able to provide support caring and supervision like friends or teachers
- Create a plan with the parent/caregiver that these supports are available when needed

2 = Limited supervision and/or assistance available from family/ caregiver, friends/peers, teachers, and/or community social networks

- Complete actions under Risk Level 1
- Look for alternative supports like after-school care or community activities

3 = No effective supervision and/or assistance available from family/ caregiver, friends/peers, teachers, and/or community social networks at any time

- Complete actions under Risk Level 2
- Get permission to speak with extended family to ascertain their ability to support the patient
- Work with school and social services to see what programs might be available to address the patient's need for additional emotional support

School and Community Participation

0 = Attending school regularly, achieving and participating well, and actively engaged in extracurricular school or community activities (e.g., sports, clubs, hobbies, religious groups)

- No action required.

1 = Average of 1 day of school missed/week and/or minor disruptions in achievement and behavior with few extracurricular activities

- Discover the reason for missed school days
- Strategize with parent/caregiver on how to prevent missed school days
- Work with parent/guardian and patient to learn what the child is interested in—hobbies, sports, games, etc.
- Encourage parent/guardian to connect patient to activates

2 = Average of 2 days or more of school missed/week and/or moderate disruption in achievement or behavior with resistance to extracurricular activities

- Complete actions under Risk Level 1
- Contact patient's school to help facilitate parent/guardian communication with teachers and school counselors to develop plan to improve attendance, performance, and participation

3 = Truant or school nonattendance with no extracurricular activities and no community connections

- Complete actions under Risk Levels 1 and 2 with plan for urgent implementation

H

ICM-CAG Scoring Sheet

Date:	HEALTH RISKS AND HEALTH NEEDS						
Name:	HISTORICAL		CURRENT STATE		VULNERABILITY		
Total Score =	Complexity Item	Score	Complexity Item	Score	Complexity Item	Score	
Biological Domain	Chronic Illness		Symptom Severity/ Impairment		Complications and Life Threat		
	Diagnostic Difficulty		Adherence Ability				
Psychological Domain	Barriers to Coping		Resistance to Treatment		Mental Health Threat		
	Mental Health History		Mental Health Symptoms				
Social Domain	Job and Leisure		Residential Stability		Social Vulnerability		
	Relationships		Social Support				
Health System Domain	Access to Care		Getting Needed Services		Health System Deterrents		
	Treatment Experience		Provider Collaboration				
Comments							
(Enter pertinent information about the reason for the score of each complexity item here, (e.g.,.poor patient adherence, death in family with stress to patient, non-evidence-based treatment of migraine.)							

Scoring System
Green   0 = no need to act
Yellow   1 = mild risk and need for monitoring or prevention
Orange 2 = moderate risk and need for action or development of intervention plan
Red   3 = severe risk and need for immediate action or immediate intervention plan

Note: Permission for re-use must be obtained from the authors by contacting ICM@cmsa.org.

PIM-CAG Scoring Sheet

Date:	HEALTH RISKS AND HEALTH NEEDS					
Name:	HISTORICAL		CURRENT STATE		VULNERABILITY	
Total Score =	Complexity Item	Score	Complexity Item	Score	Complexity Item	Score
Biological Domain	Chronic Illness		Symptom Severity/ Impairment		Complications and Life Threat	
	Diagnostic Difficulty		Adherence Ability			
Psychological Domain	Barriers to Coping		Resistance to Treatment		Learning and/ or Mental Health Threat	
	Mental Health History		Mental Health Symptoms			
	Cognitive Development					
	Adverse Developmental Events					
Social Domain	Learning Ability		Residential Stability		Family/School/ Social System Vulnerability	
	Family and Social Relationships		Child/ Adolescent Support System			
	Caregiver/ Parent Health and Function		Caregiver/ Family Support			
			School and Community Participation			

(continued)

Date:	HEALTH RISKS AND HEALTH NEEDS					
Name:	HISTORICAL		CURRENT STATE		VULNERABILITY	
Total Score =	Complexity Item	Score	Complexity Item	Score	Complexity Item	Score
Health System Domain	Access to Care		Getting Needed Services		Health System Deterrents	
	Treatment Experience		Provider Collaboration			
Comments						

Scoring System
Green   0 = no need to act
Yellow   1 = mild risk and need for monitoring or prevention
Orange   2 = moderate risk and need for action or development of intervention plan
Red   3 = severe risk and need for immediate action or immediate intervention plan

Note: Permission for re-use must be obtained from the authors by contacting ICM@cmsa.org.

●●●●

Definition of Terms

Acuity: Related to the recentness with which an illness has shown presentation or increase in symptoms.

Age of consent: The minimum age at which a person is considered to be legally competent of consenting to sexual acts.

Care management: For purposes of this manual, this term is intended to encompass all forms of management activity, including health coaching (wellness), employee assistance, disability management and workers' compensation management, disease management, and case management. It is considered synonymous with "health management."

Case management extender: Nonclinical staff who support case managers in completing care coordination activities that do not require clinical intervention as well as working directly with patients who may need only social support and do not need clinical interventions, and can encourage, support, and coordinate preventative services for patients needing to complete.

Child abuse and neglect: Any type of cruelty inflicted on a child, including mental abuse, physical harm, neglect, and sexual abuse or exploitation.

Clinician: Any clinical-based health care professional who assists the patient in receiving interventions that will lead to better clinical outcomes, such as nurse, social worker, counselor, pharmacist, doctor, and so forth; or in a clinical helper role, such as treating practitioner, case or disease manager, therapy provider, medication advisors, and so forth. Hospital or health plan administrators are not clinicians since they are not clinical-based health care professionals. Utilization managers, even though they are most often clinical-based health care professionals, are not clinicians since they are not functioning in a helper role.

Comorbidity: The occurrence of two or more illnesses or conditions in the same patient.

Complexity: The combination of biological, psychological, social, and health system circumstances that creates barriers to improvement, making it difficult for a person with illness to regain or stabilize health.

Cross-disciplinary roles: The primary case manager works with the member in all areas that impact health by becoming familiar with conditions less familiar.

Evidence-based practice (EBP): Integrating clinical expertise with the best available external clinical evidence from systematic research.

Generalized anxiety disorder-7 (GAD-7): Standardized symptom scale for anxiety.

Health complexity: May include the presence of both medical and behavioral conditions, multiple chronic illnesses, the presence of social concerns, poor access to needed care and services, impairments or disabilities, and financial concerns.

Individualized care: Connecting a health professional with a general understanding of illnesses, treatments, the health system, and factors that create barriers to improvement, such as a case manager, to a patient/client with persistent health problems in an attempt to actively and personally assist him or her stabilize or return to health over a period of days to years. This form of care is patient-centered, focusing on all complexity domains, with an outcome orientation.

Integrated behavioral health benefits: In the context of this manual, it refers to the process by which a medical health plan not only owns behavioral health management and payment but also makes it a part of the physical health benefits and adjudication process.

Integrated care: For the purpose of this manual, this term applies to the availability of coordinated health services from all complexity domains (biological, psychological, social, and health system) without hassle or impediment.

Integrated case management: Follows Case Management Society of America's Standards of Practice for guidance and accountability in case management practice, and is designed to impact individuals with health complexity by a single point of contact, or primary case manager through a multidimensional approach.

Long-term disability: Generally employees with permanent conditions, requiring time away from work for more than 6 months and little likelihood of improvement; when long-term disability is supported by a documentable medical condition, (a) the disabled person is paid a percentage of his or her prior salary, (b) he or she must document persistence of disabling signs and symptoms over time, and (c) the employer has no obligation to take the person back to his or her prior position (unemployed—disabled).

Mental health parity: Under the Affordable Care Act (ACA) passed in 2010, behavioral health services were included as one of the 10 essential benefits, meaning, insurers were required to cover mental health services equally to that of medical services.

Motivational interviewing: A person-centered counseling style for addressing the common problem of ambivalence about change.

Patient Health Questionnaire-9 (PHQ-9): Standardized symptom scale for depression.

Population health management: The health outcomes of a group of individuals including the distribution of such outcomes within the group to improve the health of an entire human population by reducing health inequities or disparities due to social determinants of health.

Professional case manager: Performs the primary functions of assessment, planning, facilitation, coordination, monitoring, evaluation, and advocacy.

Severity: The seriousness of an illness; this is a component of complexity.

Shared decision making: A process by which a health care choice is made by the patient (or significant others, or both) together with one or more health care professionals.

Short-term disability (STD): Time-limited illness in an employee that prevents his or her ability to work (usually 6 months or less); during this time the employee retains his or her job, is paid during the time away from work, and cannot be fired or permanently replaced (employed—disabled).

Transference: The patient's emotional reaction to a clinician, which is hypothesized to emanate from relationships with others (psychiatric jargon).

Utilization management: The practice of approving or denying payment for services based on the presence of covered benefit or medical necessity; this is *not* considered a form.

Warm transfer: The enrollment specialist keeps the patient on the line while the case manager who will be assuming responsibility for the case is brought on the line, personally introduced, and a short summary of the situation is given.

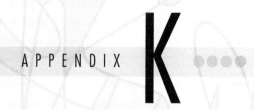
Abbreviations

AA	Alcoholics Anonymous
ABI/TBI	acute brain injury/traumatic brain injury
ACE	angiotensin-converting enzyme
ADHD	attention deficit hyperactivity disorder
ADL	activities of daily living
BI	brain injury
CAG	Complexity Assessment Grid
CBT	cognitive behavioral therapy
CCM	certified case manager
CHF	congestive heart failure
CM	case management
CMSA	Case Management Society of America
CNS	central nervous system
COPD	chronic obstructive pulmonary disease
CPT	current procedural terminology
CT	computed tomography
CVD	cardiovascular disease
DM	disease management
DME	durable medical equipment
DSM-5	*Diagnostic and Statistical Manual of Mental Disorders*, 5th edition
Dx	diagnosis

(*continued*)

ED	emergency department
EEG	electroencephalogram
EKG	electrocardiogram
FEV_1	forced expiratory volume in 1 second
GAD-7	Generalized Anxiety Disorder Symptom Scale
GP	general practitioner
HbA1c	hemoglobin A1c
HEDIS	Healthcare Effectiveness Data and Information Set
HIV	human immunodeficiency virus
HTN	hypertension
IADL	instrumental activities of daily living
ICD-10	*International Classification of Disease,* 10th edition
ICM-CAG	Integrated Case Management Complexity Assessment Grid
IM-CAG	INTERMED-Complexity Assessment Grid
INF	infection
INTERMED	original name for the European version of the IM-CAG
IT	information technology
LOS	length of stay
MH	mental health
MH/SUD	mental health/substance use disorder
MI	motivational interviewing
NAMI	National Alliance for Mental Illness
NCQA	National Committee for Quality Assurance
NIH	National Institutes of Health
NQF	National Quality Forum
PC	primary care
PCMH	patient-centered medical home
PCP	primary care physician
PH	physical health

(continued)

PHI	personal health information
PHQ-2	Patient Health Questionnaire-2
PHQ-9	Patient Health Questionnaire-9
PIM-CAG	pediatric version of the INTERMED-Complexity Assessment Grid
PTSD	posttraumatic stress disorder
Rx	prescription
SDM	shared decision making
SDOH	social determinants of health
SMI	serious mental illness
SNRI	serotonin–norepinephrine reuptake inhibitor
SPMI	serious and persistent mental illness
SSRI	selective serotonin reuptake inhibitor (class of antidepressant and antianxiety agents)
SUD	substance use disorder
TTM	transtheoretical model
UM	utilization management
URAC	Utilization Review Accreditation Commission

L

Suggested Scripted Interview Questions

Introduction and General Life Questions

"Hello Mr./Mrs./Ms. _____, my name is _____ and I am a nurse/social worker case manager from _____. I am reaching out to see if I can be of any assistance to you."

"Is it alright to ask a few questions so that I can get to know you before we focus on your current health situation?"

If the patient answers yes, "Are you comfortable telling me a little about yourself? I'm interested in knowing how you spend your days; do have any hobbies or interests?"

If the patient is hesitant, try these questions:

"Do you work outside the home? If so, what kind of work do you do?"

"Do you have any difficulties meeting your financial obligations like rent, mortgage, utilities, food, medications, and so on?"

"Do you take care of anyone beside yourself? Children, parents, other relatives, neighbors, etc.?"

"Do you have any difficulties taking care of yourself (bathing, cooking, housekeeping)? If so, who helps you?"

"Who are the people who support you when you need help?"

"Whom do you call when a crisis occurs?"

"How do you like to spend your free time?"

Physical Health Questions

"Tell me how your _____ is affecting you today."

"Tell me about the physical illnesses you have had and how they have affected your life."

"What kind of symptoms are you having?"

"Were they difficult to diagnose? If so, how long did it take? Were many tests done?"

"What kind of treatment has the doctor prescribed? Has the treatment been helpful, effective?"

"Is it difficult for you to follow the doctor's orders? If so, why?"

"Do the symptoms interfere with your life? If so, how?"

Emotional Health Questions

"Do you ever feel worried, tense, and/or forgetful?"

"If yes, how often?"

"Has your physical health affected your emotions?"

"Have you had any mental health problems in the past? If so, tell me about them."

"Have you ever been hospitalized for a mental health condition? If so, why and for how long?"

"Have you ever received treatment for a mental or behavioral condition? If so, what kind of treatment?"

"Have you ever had difficulty following prescribed treatment for a mental or behavioral condition? If so, what kind of difficulty?"

"Are you receiving any treatment at present? If so, what has been prescribed and is it helping?"

"Do any emotional feelings interfere with your ability to work or do the things you like to do?"

Health System Questions

"Do you ever have trouble getting the care you need?"

"Do you have adequate coverage for your health care needs? If not, what care are you unable to access?"

"Do you have a primary doctor? Are you able to get appointments when you need them?"

"If no, have you had difficulty finding a trusted doctor? If so, is that something I can help with?"

"Do you see any specialists? If so, for what reasons?"

"Do you prefer a doctor who speaks your first language? Have you been able to find such a doctor?"

"If no, would you like to have a translator present for your appointments?"

"Do you have any cultural or religious practices that interfere with the prescribed treatment? If so, can you tell me about them?"

"Do you have any trouble paying for medical care?"

"Are you able to get to your appointments? Do you need assistance with transportation?"

"Do you live some distance from your providers? Would you like help in finding providers closer to where you live?"

"If you see multiple doctors, do you know if they communicate regarding your care?"

Personal Information Questions

"Do you smoke or use any tobacco products?"

"Are you interested in quitting?"

"Do you use any prescription painkillers? If yes, what kind and how often do you take them?"

"Do you use any illegal substances? If so, which ones and how often do you use them? Are you interested in treatment for substance use?"

"Do you drink alcohol? If yes, how often? Do you believe that alcohol is a problem for you? If yes, are you interested in treatment?"

"What are your biggest concerns right now?"

"In the next 3 months, what would you like to work on related to your health?"

"What would you like to be able to do that you cannot do right now (exercise, go to church, play with grandchildren, etc.)?

"What things are important to you that we did not discuss?"

Index